"Press to shock," the machine intoned. "Press to shock."

"Everyone clear!" I yelled. When everyone was away from the table, I pressed the shock button. The machine delivered a 200-joule jolt of electricity through Tony's heart. Steve pressed his fingers against Tony's neck and palpated for a carotid pulse. "No pulse."

"We better continue CPR and reevaluate in the rig," I said.

The four of us quickly wheeled Tony to the ambulance and lifted him in. We prepared to continue CPR as Marge got into the driver's seat. I felt for Tony's carotid artery and was amazed to find it pulsing strongly. "There's a pulse." I leaned my ear to his mouth. "Yeah," I shouted. "He's breathing."

I called the hospital and told them what had happened, informing them we would be arriving in about five minutes. When I returned my attention to Tony, he had opened his eyes. "Hey there, Tony," I said. "Nice to have you back. . . ."

DIAL 911

Joan E. Lloyd
Edwin B. Herman

IVY BOOKS • NEW YORK

Ivy Books
Published by Ballantine Books
Copyright © 1995 by Joan E. Lloyd and Edwin B. Herman

Library of Congress Catalog Card Number: 95-94544

ISBN 0-8041-1315-7

Manufactured in the United States of America

First Edition: November 1995

10 9 8 7 6 5 4 3 2 1

This book is dedicated to
Norman and Zet, David and Pauline.

Now we know how
difficult
and wonderful
it is to be a parent.

Chapter 1

Tony Piamonte awoke feeling poorly. "I really feel punk," he told his wife over breakfast. "Must be coming down with the flu."

"How punk?" his wife, Angela, asked.

"Oh, I don't know." He sipped his coffee but ignored the bacon and eggs his wife had prepared. "My stomach's upset. I feel like I have a gas bubble lodged right here." He pointed to the center of his chest. "I feel a bit light-headed and, I don't know, breathless."

"This is pretty sudden. You seemed to be fine when we went to bed."

"It woke me up about four in the morning."

"Did you take anything?"

"Yes, dear," he snapped. "I took some Maalox, like a good boy. It did nothing at all."

"Don't get nasty with me," Angela said. "That's not like you either."

"I'm sorry," he said, genuinely apologetic. "I'm just a bit jumpy. This pain is starting to get to me." He took another sip of coffee.

"I think you should go see Dr. Parks."

"Doctors. Bah. They'll tell me to take Alka-Seltzer and then charge me fifty dollars." Tony rubbed the heel of his hand up and down his breastbone and grimaced.

"Dear," Angela said firmly, "I'll get the car out of the garage and drive you."

After a brief argument, Angela prevailed. They drove to the doctor's office and were waiting when Dr. Parks

1

arrived. The doctor motioned Tony into one of the back examining rooms and sent a nurse to get a set of vitals.

The insistent beep ... beep ... beep of my pager interrupted my thoughts. "Fairfax police to the ambulance corps. A full crew is needed for a call at the professional building in town, Dr. Llewellan's office, for a man who needs to be transported to the hospital. All available members please call in."

A transport, I thought as I tried to resist the pager, assuming that someone else would respond. I was writing a book proposal and I had a deadline to meet. Like most of the other emergency medical technicians who ride with the Fairfax Volunteer Ambulance Corps, I don't like to do transports. They take a lot of time and, since we normally have little to do for our patient except make small talk, they're usually boring. I continued to peck away at my word processor and hoped that others would call in.

Thirty seconds later the pagers sounded again. "A full crew is still needed for this call at Dr. Llewellan's office. Please call in."

By the third page, the police dispatcher was sounding desperate. I couldn't, in good conscience, let him call Prescott, our neighboring corps, for mutual aid. Calling Prescott would substantially delay the response and take a Prescott rig away from its own district. Reluctantly I phoned police headquarters. "This is Joan Lloyd. I'll respond to the scene."

"Thanks, Joan," Greg Horvath said. "Marge Talbot just called in and she is picking up the rig. Steve Nesbitt will meet you at the scene. He said that he just got out of the shower so he'll be delayed a few minutes." As I trotted to my car, I heard Greg page out to inform FVAC members that the call was covered.

Dr. Llewellan's office is only a short distance from my condo so I arrived minutes before the ambulance. As I pulled into the overcrowded parking area, my radio came alive. "Fairfax police to units responding to Dr. Llewellan's office. The patient is now reported to be in cardiac arrest. Code 99—CPR in progress."

I scooted my car into an almost-filled no-parking area and sprinted into the doctor's office. "Where?" I puffed.

The nurse motioned me into a back examining room. As I approached, I heard the familiar chant "One and two and three and four and five," then a pause. As I entered, Dr. Llewellan, a rotund, fatherly-looking man with a wonderful bedside manner, was blowing air into the patient's mouth through a simple face shield. His new associate, Dr. Parks, stood on the rung of the exam table doing chest compressions.

"We need a defibrillator," Dr. Parks yelled.

"I arrived before the rig," I said. "It'll be here momentarily." I looked at the patient, a man who seemed to be in his mid-fifties, dressed in a brown-and-green-patterned pullover sweater and brown slacks. "Do either of you need me to take over?"

"I'm fine," Dr. Parks said, and Dr. Llewellan shook his head.

"Okay. Where's a scissors so I can cut open his sweater?"

"On the counter," Dr. Llewellan said.

As I retrieved the scissors, I looked at Dr. Llewellan and asked, "What happened?"

"He's my patient," Dr. Parks said. "He came in with his wife first thing this morning complaining of indigestion. I gather he wasn't going to come in at all but his wife insisted." As he talked and continued his rhythmic compressions, I cut up the front of the man's sweater around the doctor's hands. "We put him in here," Dr. Parks continued, "and as the nurse was taking his blood pressure, he suddenly collapsed. He had no pulse and was not breathing so we began CPR."

"45–01 on location," my portable radio announced. I keyed the mike. "CPR in progress. Bring the mega-duffel and the defibrillator, stat."

"10–4, Joan," Marge said. "And Steve's just pulling up."

Marge and Steve arrived in the exam room and we went to work. Steve took the oxygen cylinder from the megaduffel and hooked it up to a bag valve mask so he could better ventilate the patient. After he inserted an oral airway to keep the man's tongue from obstructing his airway, he held the mask pressed against the victim's face. Dr. Llewellan squeezed the bag to deliver 800 cc doses of pure oxygen into the unconscious man's lungs, while Dr. Parks continued compressions.

Marge opened the defibrillator case and pulled out two six-inch-diameter round pads and removed the backing. Using the peel-and-stick adhesive, she attached one just beneath the patient's right collarbone and another against his left lower ribs.

"His name?" I asked.

"Tony Piamonte."

As I withdrew the two leads from their pocket in the defibrillator case, I continued, "Any history?"

"None that we know of," Dr. Parks answered.

"He's been a patient of ours for about ten years," Dr. Llewellan added, "and there's been nothing unusual until this."

Holding the defibrillator in one arm, I snapped the leads onto the pads and opened the monitor. "Stop CPR." Everyone moved away from the table. "I'm reading coarse v-fib," I said, looking at the screen while holding the defibrillator as still as possible in order to get an accurate reading. Ventricular fibrillation is disorganized cardiac muscle activity that won't pump blood effectively. Dr. Parks came around behind me and nodded. I quickly pressed the Analyze button. Almost immediately I heard the characteristic whine as the machine began to charge, allowing us to deliver a shock to the heart muscle.

Suddenly I realized that I was still holding the defibrillator, and I could see no place to put it down. I couldn't hold it as it shocked, and the leads wouldn't reach the floor or any of the tables or counters. With no other choice, I placed the machine, about the size of the Manhattan Yellow Pages, on the patient's thighs. I prepared to catch it if it fell as Tony's body reacted to the shock.

"Press to shock," the machine intoned. "Press to shock."

"Everyone clear!" I yelled. When everyone was away from the table, I pressed the shock button. The machine delivered a 200-joule jolt of electricity through Tony's heart. As the machine slipped from his body, I caught it and pressed the Analyze button again. "I see what looks like a very slow, viable rhythm. The machine won't deliver another shock."

"Are you sure?" Dr. Parks asked.

The defibrillator's screen displayed the message "No shock indicated." The machine is programmed to recognize cardiac rhythms. Since we're EMTs and can't give drugs, the defibrillator will only let us shock those we can help directly, v-tach and v-fib. And the rhythm the machine was sensing was neither ventricular tachycardia, extremely rapid heartbeat, nor ventricular fibrillation, useless, disorganized heart muscle activity.

"Does he have a pulse?" I asked Steve, who stood at Tony's head.

Steve pressed his fingers against Tony's neck and palpated for a carotid pulse. "No pulse."

"We better continue CPR and reevaluate in the rig," I said.

Marge took over compressions and Dr. Parks joined Steve on ventilations. "I'll go along," the doctor said. "Jake," he yelled to Dr. Llewellan, "get me an IV setup. I can start a line KVO in the ambulance." He turned to us. "KVO," he explained. "To keep the vein open. That will make it easier for the emergency room staff to give meds when we get there."

The four of us wheeled Tony to the ambulance, stopping twice for cycles of CPR, and lifted him in. I climbed around to the jumpseat near Tony's head, and Steve and Dr. Parks sat at his side on the crew bench. We prepared to continue CPR as Marge got into the driver's seat.

"Give us a minute," I yelled to her, as I rechecked Tony's heart rhythm on the monitor. "I see a normal sinus rhythm," I said, showing the monitor to Dr. Parks.

"So do I," he agreed.

The fact that the monitor showed electrical rhythm didn't mean Tony's heart was beating. I felt for his carotid artery and was amazed to find it pulsing strongly. "There's a pulse." I leaned my ear to his mouth. "Yeah," I shouted. "He's breathing."

I leaned through the window to the cab. "Let's go, Marge. He's breathing and has a pulse but he's still unconscious and needs medical attention stat."

I leaned over and yelled into Tony's ear. "You're doing good, Tony. Hang in there. Stay with us." Even while unconscious, patients may be able to hear.

Dr. Parks felt for Tony's radial pulse and, after a moment's concentration, said, "Pulse is good, about 60. You must have a BP of at least 80 systolic to get a radial pulse."

Marge pulled into traffic, siren screaming. "Nice job, guys," I said. Tony moaned and gagged, starting to thrash his head around. "It's okay, Tony," I said as I quickly removed the airway from his throat. "We're taking good care of you." I saw Dr. Parks tapping the crook of his elbow so I said, "Dr. Parks is going to start an IV so you'll feel a little stick."

I called the hospital and told them what had happened, informing them we would be arriving in about five minutes. When I returned my attention to Tony, he had opened his eyes. "Hey there, Tony," I said. "Nice to have you back."

* * *

Tony Piamonte stayed in the hospital for about two weeks. Then, almost a month later, Tony and his wife and daughter, the ambulance crew, Drs. Parks and Llewellan, and two of the nurses from their office got together for a celebratory lunch at our local watering hole. "You know," Tony said, "when I woke up in the ambulance everyone was so happy, I thought I had won the lottery."

I see Tony and his family around town from time to time and we reminisce about that morning, now almost three years ago. It's quite a feeling for me to see someone who might not be alive now had it not been for me and my crew and the doctors.

Ed and I made a special trip to Tony's house when our first book, *Rescue Alert*, came out. We gave him a signed copy, especially inscribed:

"To someone who now has two birthdays."

My name is Joan Lloyd. I have two grown daughters and, as of this writing, 1.3 grandchildren. In the nine years that I've been an EMT (emergency medical technician), Tony Piamonte's recovery after his sudden-death heart attack was one of my most rewarding calls. It sounds a bit like one of the situations portrayed on the TV program *Rescue 911*: very dramatic, with a happy ending in which the victim and rescuers celebrate at a party afterward.

Most of our calls, and indeed most of the stories in this book, are not as dramatic as this one, and many do not have the traditional happy ending. Furthermore, we seldom become good friends with the people we treat. This is the real world, not the world of television.

We, as ambulance personnel, are privy to information that most people wouldn't know: intimate and sometimes confidential details of life and, occasionally, death. Ed and I do not want to hurt or embarrass anyone, patient or rescuer, family or bystander. Therefore, the stories you are about to read, although based on the true events, have been fictionalized. We have changed the names and places to protect everyone involved. So welcome to the Fairfax Volunteer Ambulance Corps and the fictional town of Fairfax, a bedroom community about fifty miles from a large city.

While Ed and I have been a part of many of the stories you are about to read, some are based on experiences of friends and colleagues. We've also gotten wonderful tales from readers of our first book. Emergency workers from all over the country have written to tell us their own, personal stories, and a few of them are included here.

Emergency medicine is a constantly changing field. What is common practice at one time in one area of the country may be different at another time in another place. As Ed and I write this book, our protocols regarding the MAST, a device you'll read about later, as well as several other procedures, are changing. The methods used by the emergency medical personnel in this book were correct at the time the story occurred.

Emergency medicine, like other fields, has its jargon, and we've tried to explain each term or acronym the first time it's used. You'll find a glossary at the back of this book listing and explaining many of these words and phrases.

Those of you who have read *Rescue Alert* will notice that Ed has recently joined the Prescott Rescue Squad, which responds to ambulance calls with paramedics as well as EMTs. EMTs splint, bandage, extricate, and defibrillate but do not do anything that invades the body. Only a paramedic, with eight hundred hours of training, can start intravenous lines, give medications, and intubate—place a tube into the patient's throat to assist breathing.

For simplicity we've reduced the number of people we work with to an unrealistically small number. Although each of the corps with which Ed and I ride has about one hundred members, Fairfax Ambulance Corps has fewer than two dozen. Likewise we mention only a few members of the police and fire departments, one emergency room doctor at Fairfax General Hospital, and a handful of nurses. These people are listed in "The Cast" at the end of this book. All the adventures you are about to read, however, are based on the real world of the emergency medical technician.

Chapter 2

My name is Ed Herman and I'm fifty-six years old. I've wanted to be involved in emergency work ever since I was a kid, but my actual involvement began only about twenty years ago in a town about five miles south of Fairfax.

Damn, I thought, today is going to be a reverse "Midas touch" day; everything I touch seems to be turning to garbage. I had forgotten to set the alarm, overslept, and, in my rush to get to work, I had dropped my juice and cut my foot on a piece of the broken glass. It had taken me ten minutes to stop the bleeding. As I drove south toward the parkway, traffic was moving at a crawl. Just as it was beginning to open up, the traffic light at Broad and First, the last one before the parkway entrance, changed in my face. I settled down to wait for the light cycle, which I knew to be a long one.

It was only 8:30 A.M. and the sun was shining brightly, but I felt like I had a rain cloud over my head. I glanced to my right and saw a couple of kids on a motorcycle approaching the intersection, a boy driving and a girl behind him, her arms around his waist and her red hair streaming behind her. Boy, that's the way to travel, I thought enviously.

I had ridden a motorcycle as a youth, all the way to Mexico, with a girl and an assortment of camping gear on the back of my 90 cc Honda. It was wonderful, but as I grew older I started to feel that riding a motorcycle was like playing Russian roulette. The kind of minor accident that might dent a fender on a car could kill me on a bike. So I had finally gotten rid of my little red Honda. But sometimes I missed it a lot, especially while sitting in traffic on a beautiful morning like this.

As I gazed at the approaching bike, I suddenly heard the blare of a horn behind me. Glancing up at the rearview mirror, I saw a car with flashing headlights and a blue strobe on its roof coming up rapidly behind me on the right shoulder of the road. The car sped past me and, without slowing, charged through the red light and into the intersection. There was a short squeal of brakes and a crash of metal against metal. I stared in disbelief at the sight of the two kids sailing in an almost graceful arc through the air and landing about thirty feet away, at the far side of the intersection.

I pulled my car over to the side of the road, jumped out, and ran across the intersection, almost getting hit by an oncoming car. The boy lay on his back in the grass shrieking and clutching his groin. The girl had landed facedown across a low hedge. She was quiet. I looked at the screaming boy. Surely he needed help more than the girl. But at that time I had no EMS training, no idea of what to do.

I went over to the boy. "Don't worry," I said. "You'll be okay."

"Carol," he shrieked. "Carol, are you all right?" His terrified eyes caught mine. "Is Carol okay?" he cried. "Please, see if she's all right."

I walked over to where Carol lay slumped over the hedge. Her head was hanging down and although she was softly groaning, she seemed to be unconscious. Blood dripped slowly from her mouth and ran down her arm from a deep gash just above her elbow. I knew she was badly injured, maybe dying, but there was nothing that I knew to do. It was the most helpless feeling that I had ever had in my life.

The boy was trying to get up. I knew that it was important to keep him from moving. With relief I realized that there was something I could do. I went back to him. "Don't move," I said. "You've got to lie still."

"I've got to help Carol. Is she all right?"

"Yes," I lied. "She's fine. Someone is taking care of her."

The boy managed to turn his head until he could see Carol's limp form. "You're lying. She's dead," he shrieked, becoming increasingly agitated. "I killed her." He tried to get up but fell back in pain.

"She's doing okay. She's not dead. She's breathing."

"You're lying to me. She's dead." He kept struggling with me. "Carol, Carol! I'm sorry. I have to tell her that. I have to say good-bye. I have to be with her."

I had only limited success keeping him quiet. I knew that moving could complicate his injuries, but he was determined to talk to his girlfriend. Although other people stopped to help, no one knew what to do and Carol lay alone, slumped over the hedge.

I stayed with the boy for what seemed like hours until the local volunteer ambulance arrived. The EMTs worked on both patients, calmly and efficiently examining, treating, and immobilizing them. As the ambulance rolled away, siren wailing and lights flashing, I had no idea whether the kids would live or die. I didn't even know the boy's name.

As I think back now, I realize that that was the day I decided that I would never again be in such a helpless position.

The following Saturday afternoon I walked through the open bay doors, past the two ambulances, into the headquarters of the Fairfax Volunteer Ambulance Corps, FVAC. At the side of the ambulance bay was a door with a sign that read ABANDON HOPE YE WHO ENTER HERE. I knocked on it and a voice called out, "Come on in."

I walked into a rather messy kitchen with a small table, around which sat three people playing cards: a middle-aged couple and a teenage girl, all wearing white uniform shirts. The couple had EMT symbols on their right sleeves. Above the left shirt pocket of each uniform was a blue, red, and gold patch: swords crossed in front of a burning candle. I found out later that it stood for the ambulance corps' efforts to defend the candle of life.

"Hi, I'm Ed," I said.

"Hi," the man said, extending his hand. "I'm Hank and this is my wife, Paula. What can we do for you?"

"I was wondering how I can get the training that I would need to become a member of the ambulance corps."

"You don't need any training to join us," Hank replied. "New members are always welcome. You start as a probationary member and you can train while you ride the ambulance. We use probies to fetch and carry equipment and sometimes as wheel chocks for the ambulances." He chuckled and the girl at the end of the table made a rude noise.

"I thought you had to be an EMT," I said.

"Ultimately, you have to become a state-certified EMT," he explained, "and I think you learn best both by studying and by riding with us."

"Is it expensive?" I asked, settling down in an empty chair.

"We reimburse you once you pass the course."

"Is it hard?"

Paula answered. "It's about one hundred and ten hours. It's demanding, but if you ride and take the course, you'll do fine."

"Then what?"

"Once you have completed your EMT training, you become a regular member." Hank opened a drawer, pulled out a sheet of paper, and handed it to me. "Here's an application form. As soon as you fill it out and return it to us, our membership committee chairman will get in touch with you."

"By the way," Paula said, "the kid over there is Rosemary. She rides with us as a youth group cadet and she's better than some of the old-timers. Coffee?" she offered.

As I took the mug of dark brew Paula handed me, out of the corner of my eye I glimpsed a familiar-looking small, furry black-and-white animal slink around the corner of a doorway leading out of the kitchen. Hank laughed as he noticed my face drain of color as I stared at the spot where the animal had suddenly appeared and just as suddenly vanished.

"Don't worry about Sunshine." He chuckled. "She's had her scent glands removed. Paula and I have had her for five years. We found her as a little skunklet. Her mother must have abandoned her or been killed by a car so we raised her. She's shy with strangers, but by the time you're a regular member she'll be climbing into your lap. She usually lives with us and visits here while we're riding, but our grandchildren are visiting for a week and she's terrified of them so we brought her to FVAC for the week. She knows everyone here and she's quite comfortable."

"I'm sure she's a great pet," I muttered, unconvinced, imagining a skunk climbing into my lap.

We had been talking for about an hour, when the harsh blare of a klaxon startled me so that I spilled my second cup of coffee. The radio in the communications cubicle occupying a corner of the kitchen came to life.

"Fairfax Police to Fairfax Ambulance."

Paula calmly got up and spoke into a microphone. "Fairfax Ambulance on. Go ahead Fairfax Police."

"The ambulance is needed to respond to a 10–2 at the intersection of Springfield and Main. 45–18 is at the scene and advises you respond 10–15."

I was baffled. That communication wasn't in any language I understood.

Sensing my confusion, Paula said, "We'll have to ask you to leave the building now. We're responding to a

10–2, a personal injury automobile accident. But one of our members, radio number 45–18, is at the scene and has advised us that it's not serious and we don't have to use our lights and siren."

As I stood outside the FVAC building holding the membership application in my hand and watching the ambulance roll out of its bay and down the street, it seemed that I was about to begin something I had always wanted to do but never knew it.

I rode with Hank and Paula often until they left the corps a few years later. Rosemary Harper is now the head emergency room nurse at Fairfax General.

Looking back now, I feel sad when I think of how helpless I was at the scene of that motorcycle accident twenty years ago, but at least I knew that an injured person must be kept still and not moved. Since that time, I haven't felt helpless at the scene of any medical emergency. I've felt sad, frustrated, angry, even hostile, but never helpless. There's always something I can do, anything from stopping bleeding to setting up road flares to warn traffic. Even in nonmedical emergencies my training and experience have enabled me to act in a calm and rational manner—to be effective without endangering my own health or safety.

I have also learned that volunteers, like the one that hit that motorcycle twenty years ago, even with lights flashing on their personal vehicles, have no right to violate traffic laws, much less speed into intersections and endanger life and property. And I realize that by lying to the motorcycle driver, I made him more anxious, not less. So now I never, never lie to my patients.

Chapter 3

In Fairfax and its surrounding towns, an ambulance call is classified by the emergency services as either a 10–3 or a 10–2. A medical emergency is called a 10–3: a call for a person feeling ill, having difficulty breathing, and/or having chest pains. When we get dispatched for a 10–3, we respond and check the patient's condition; in Fairfax, since we do not have paramedics available, as Ed does when he rides with Prescott, we make the patient as comfortable as we can, give oxygen, and transport him or her to the hospital. Often, the most important treatment we can offer is psychological first aid. Once patients realize that we are going to make them comfortable and get them to the hospital quickly, they usually relax, easing the stress on their body. This alone often improves their condition.

The second type of call is a personal injury automobile accident, also called a PIAA or a 10–2. Although similar, each call for a PIAA has an individual character.

Ed was unavailable so I was riding midnight to 6 A.M. with Stephanie DiMartino and Bob Fiorella. Stephanie and I were riding from home and Bob was sleeping at headquarters. It was almost 2:00 A.M. and I was sound asleep when the phone rang. The police dispatcher told me that there had been a PIAA on Route 541 near the reservoir. I absorbed the information and was fully awake, dressed, and out of the house in less than two minutes. Since it was mid-October I had to take an extra minute to scrape some accumulated early-fall ice from my windshield.

I arrived at the scene just as the rig, with Bob driving, pulled to a stop. Stephanie drove up only fifteen seconds later.

Three police cars had Route 541 blocked in both directions. I surveyed the scene and saw a late-model Ford crumpled against the guard rail that separated the roadway from the wooded area beside the water. Only one car. That was good news.

Fairfax police officer Merve Berkowitz ran up to the three of us. "Damnedest thing," Merve said. "A deer must have jumped at the wrong moment and ended up going through the rear side window. The poor animal's in the backseat, all busted up, thrashing around and screaming." He shuddered. "I never heard a deer scream."

"How about the driver?" Stephanie asked.

"He's got left arm and leg injuries and is complaining of neck and back pain. He's stuck in there good so I've called for the jaws." The fire department would bring the jaws of life, or Hurst Tool, to cut, pry, pull, push—do whatever was necessary to get our patient out of the car quickly but without causing additional injury.

Just to be sure, I asked, "Only the driver in the car? No one else was with him? No other cars involved?"

"Just the one patient," Merve answered.

As the four of us trotted toward the car, Stephanie asked, "Can we get behind the driver to stabilize his head?"

"Not yet," Merve answered. "The deer's too dangerous for anyone to climb around in the backseat."

I saw that two other officers were using their portable radios to talk to the police dispatcher. "We'll shoot the deer in a minute," Merve continued, "and you may want to be in with the driver when we do."

"The deer's in that bad shape?"

"I'm afraid so. Even if we had time, what with the driver and all, I don't think the animal control officer could do anything better."

Oh, shit, I thought. They'll have to shoot the poor thing with the driver right there. I looked at the car. The driver's door was bashed in from where the deer must have bounced against it before going through the back window. "Can I get to the front passenger seat?" I asked.

"Yeah," Merve answered, "I guess so. We've got the door on that side open. We just can't get the driver out yet. He's entangled in the pedals and the driver's door is pressed against his left side."

As I headed around to the passenger side of the car, Stephanie asked, "Want me to get in instead?"

"I'll do it." I knew she wanted to be with the deer and the driver as little as I did, but it was my responsibility since I was crew chief that night.

I always seem to take on the shitty jobs myself, I thought, and this is going to be one of the shittiest. I opened the passenger-side door and carefully slid into the seat, thinking that I had to avoid shaking the car so as not to increase the damage that the accident might have done to the driver's neck. What a ridiculous thought, I realized. The deer, a young one with light spots still covering its back, was kicking and struggling, shaking the car and everything in it. Its small hoofs were slashing dangerously close to the driver's head, around the driver-side headrest. I could see that the backs of both front seats were shredded. The agonized deer was making a keening sound, punctuated by bouts of heavy, panting breaths.

"My name's Joan," I told the driver, my voice soft and soothing, both for my patient and for the deer. "Just try to relax and we'll have you out of here in a few minutes." I placed my right hand gently against his forehead, pressing the back of his head against the headrest. "Try not to move," I told the man. "What's your name?"

"Eric," the man answered. "Eric Martinsen. With an 'e.' "

"Okay, Eric," I said. "Where do you hurt?"

"My left arm and hip. My foot's kind of caught under the clutch and my neck hurts. Jesus, my left side really hurts."

The police were certainly taking their time shooting this animal, I thought. What's taking so long?

My first priority was to protect the driver and myself from the hoofs of the terrified animal. But how? Still holding my patient's head, I leaned out of the passenger-side door. "Hey, someone. Can you cover us or the deer with a blanket or something? I'm worried about those hoofs."

While the crew sprinted back to the ambulance, I turned my attention back to Eric. "I'm going to let go of your head for a moment," I said over the sounds of the animal struggling in the backseat, "but please don't move." I ran my hands over his body as best I could. His lower left arm was probably broken, but his hip seemed only bruised. Since I could slide my hand down his left side from waist to knee, I realized that this part of his body would not be difficult to free from the crushed door. There was some metal wrapped around his shoulder and his feet were caught under the pedals, but those were minor problems.

"Can you wiggle your toes?" I asked.

He hesitated, then said, "Yeah. Seems okay."

"Good." I palpated the back of his neck, pressing gently against each of the cervical vertebrae I could reach. The lack of point tenderness meant that there was probably no break, but only *probably*. You can never be sure.

I can remember one driver we found walking around

after an auto accident with no pain or tenderness in his neck or back. As our protocol dictates, we collared him, did a standing takedown to a long backboard, and transported him to the hospital. We later found out that he had a C5 fracture—a broken neck. I remember my relief that we had taken such care with him. And we would take the same care with Eric. Any wrong move . . .

Having completed most of my primary assessment, I returned my palm to Eric's forehead, supporting his head against the headrest.

I saw Bob and Stephanie approach the back window and arrange a blanket over the terrified deer. Eric and I were grateful when the animal was sufficiently covered to keep the hoofs under partial control.

"How are you doing?" I asked.

"Okay, I guess. But how about getting me out of here? And what about the deer?"

"That's going to be the lousy part," I said. We both saw the lights of the approaching rescue truck. "That's the fire department," I told Eric. "They're going to set up the jaws of life and cut the car open so we can get you out. They'll have to remove the deer first though." I paused. "They're going to have to shoot him."

"Oh, God, no," Eric muttered.

"Yeah, me too," I said.

Detective Irv Greenberg, who had arrived on the scene while Bob and Stephanie were covering the deer, walked up to the driver-side window holding his revolver and nodded to me. Finally, I thought. "Hang on," I said to Eric. Bob handed a second blanket in through the passenger window and I covered Eric and myself with it. We closed our eyes and braced ourselves.

The sound of the shot was louder than I had expected and, as the deer became silent, both Eric and I let out a groan. It was done and the firefighters, wearing heavy gloves, quickly pulled the animal's body from the backseat.

The rest of the call went smoothly. With Stephanie in the backseat holding Eric's head, the firefighters took only a few minutes to cut the car away from his shoulder and feet. We immobilized him and soon were on our way to Fairfax General.

As the three of us walked out of the hospital, I looked at Stephanie's black uniform pants. They were covered with blood and fur from kneeling in the backseat of the car. Bob climbed into the driver's side of the ambulance and notified the police that we were 10–8, back in service.

Stephanie looked down at her pants and nodded sadly. "They'll wash," she said as we walked around the front of the rig.

"I guess the fawn was too young to understand cars," I said.

"Not so much young as cold," Stephanie said.

"What do you mean?"

"At this time of the year it gets warm during the day and the pavement absorbs heat while the sun shines on it. Then it cools more slowly than the grassy areas. It acts like a radiator, and a lot of animals hang around the pavement to stay warm."

"So that's why there are so many more animal road kills at this time of the year," I said as I opened the rear side door.

"And it's usually the young or the stupid who get it," Stephanie said, getting in beside Bob. "But this one was particularly rotten."

"Certainly was," I said. "But at least the driver wasn't badly hurt."

"Yeah," Stephanie said. "That's some consolation . . . I guess."

Richard Ng was driving upstate to visit his sister at just before six on a beautiful summer Sunday morning. He had left the city early to miss the traffic and was driving along the highway at over seventy miles per hour, enjoying the feel of the deserted roadway. As he rounded a bend, he saw a mother raccoon and three babies, standing calmly in the middle of the center lane. As Richard swerved to miss the animals, he lost control of his Jeep. It flipped over, rolling and bouncing into and through the woods that border that section of the parkway.

As the car came to rest on its crushed roof almost fifty feet from the pavement, Richard thanked his lucky stars that he had been wearing his lap and shoulder belts. Hanging upside-down from the harness, his head was a few inches above the Jeep's head-liner. As he tried to take a deep breath, he became aware of a sharp pain in his ribs. He felt blood trickle down, or rather up, his face from a deep cut on his chin. After freeing one arm, he used his sleeve to wipe the blood away before it ran up his nostril.

He took another minute to mentally survey his body. The Jeep's interior was crunched around his legs, and his pants were caught on twisted and torn metal in several places. Although he couldn't see either leg below midthigh, he knew from the pain that both knees were injured. He tried to wiggle his toes and, although they all moved, any movement of his left ankle caused severe pain. His upper body, head, neck, and arms felt okay. Shaken up, but not too badly. Well, he reasoned, I'm conscious and not doing too badly, all things considered, thanks to my seat belt.

He reached beside his left thigh to release his lap belt, but it wouldn't budge. Likewise, the shoulder harness wouldn't move. Richard started to squirm to free himself then stopped. "If I get loose with my legs trapped like this," he muttered, "I don't know where or how or even whether I'll fall."

He stopped trying to disentangle himself and took as deep a breath as he could. "Help!" he cried. "Get me out of here." He looked around. Trees. All he could see were trees and scrub and dirt. He couldn't see the parkway or even a lighter area in the trees surrounding him. "Help!" he cried again. "Someone help me." There was no one to hear.

One early-morning driver had seen the car swerve off the road. He drove to a phone and called the state police. Though the location was somewhat garbled, the police dispatcher had a patrol car respond to the general area. Trooper McGuire drove around looking for skid marks or wreckage. When he found nothing to indicate that there had been an accident, he reported back to headquarters that the report was unfounded.

It was almost nine when the Perillo family got on the road. They drove north toward Woodland Lake with their three children, a huge picnic lunch, and swimming gear, including inner tubes and a small inflatable rowboat.

Four-year-old Mark and his six-year-old brother, Barry, were having their usual argument in the third seat of their nine-passenger van. "You're on my side," Mark said. "Mommy, Barry's got his arm on my side of the car."

"I do not," Barry said. "And anyway, this is no-man's land. Anyone can have an arm in here." He moved his arm closer to his younger brother.

Amy, age six months, sat in her car seat with the strained expression on her face that told Helen Perillo exactly what she was doing. The fact didn't pass by the two boys either. "Yuck, Mom, Amy's making a stinky," Barry yelled. "Baby poop stinks."

"Yeah, Mom, Amy smells. She's shitting in her diaper."

"I won't have that language from you two," Helen snapped. "John," she said to her husband, "you'll have to pull over so I can change her."

Resigned to another delay, John pulled the van off onto the shoulder of the road and flipped on the four-way flashers. Helen used the middle seat to change Amy's diaper through the open side door. When she finished, she rolled up the diaper and started to put it into the diaper bag.

"You can't leave that stinky thing in here," Barry yelled. "We'll all suffocate."

"Yeah," Mark chimed in. "We'll suffolate."

"Suffo-cate," Helen corrected automatically. "And you're right. I'll get rid of this thing." Helen took the football-shaped plastic packet and walked into the woods, intending to discard it away from the road where it wouldn't be seen.

Suddenly she cocked her head to one side. What's that noise? she wondered. She stood very still, listened more closely, and thought she heard the cry again. Unwilling to look around the woods alone, she dropped the diaper and ran back to the car. Puffing, she arrived at her family. "I think I heard a man calling for help," she said to her husband. "You'd better check."

John climbed out of the driver's seat and traced his wife's path into the woods.

"Help," he heard weakly.

"Where are you?" he called.

"Here," the voice called again.

"Keep calling and I'll find you." John followed the sound and discovered the overturned Jeep with Richard still upside-down, trapped in his seat belt. "I'll get help," John said, sprinting back to the van. He bundled his family into the car and drove to the nearest phone.

When I arrived on the scene in the ambulance, with Heather and Tom Franks, two state police cars already were there. "One-car accident," a state police officer I didn't recognize said. "A Jeep and it's on its roof. The guy's hanging upside-down but we were afraid to move him without you folks here. Follow me."

Glad that my long pants and heavy socks partially protected me from brambles and deer ticks, I trekked through the underbrush, following the officer and Heather, with Tom bringing up the rear. I carried the megaduffel with its oxygen tank and trauma supplies, Heather had the KED extrication jacket, collars and straps, and Tom carried a long spineboard. The officer carried the Reeves, a slatted, rollable, plastic-covered six-foot-long stretcher with handles on each corner.

We arrived at the vehicle and I saw another state trooper leaning into the overturned Jeep. Before going any further, Heather, Tom, and I put down our gear and consulted on how we were going to handle the situation.

"Can we immobilize him in that position?" Heather asked.

I shrugged. "I don't think so. Tom?"

He looked in through the windshield. "I think we'll have to slide a board into the car, then support the guy as best we can with our hands and lower him onto it."

I took the collar bag from Heather. "Sounds like the best alternative. Let's check him out."

We questioned Richard about the accident and found that his only pains were in his ribs, knees, and ankle. "And I have a major headache from hanging upside-down all this time," he said, groaning. Tom examined his upper body from the driver's side and then put a collar around his neck, an amazingly easy task when the patient is hanging upside-down.

I climbed through the passenger window, reached up, and ran my hands the length of Richard's lower body. Awkwardly I cut hunks out of the legs of his jeans and unhooked him from some pieces of metal. Fortunately his legs were not enmeshed in the crushed metal and, except for a few deep lacerations, were not in bad shape. Although each foot was tangled around a pedal, I managed to get them both free. How we would have disentangled him if we had had to use the jaws, I have no idea.

Our full-body survey found fewer injuries than we had thought possible considering the distance the car had rolled. We slipped an air splint—an inflatable foot-shaped sleeve—onto Richard's left ankle and we bandaged both of his knees, which were cut and scraped but not broken.

Unable to do more than support Richard's body, we cut the belts and used every available hand to gently lower him onto the backboard. We strapped him down, immobilized his head, put an oxygen mask over his nose and mouth, and checked his vital signs. They were steady and strong. We set the longboard on the Reeves stretcher, then used the handles to carry Richard to the highway and the waiting ambulance.

Then we quickly transported our patient to the hospital, still amazed at his good fortune. A seat belt and luck saved him. Speed had almost killed him.

About a year ago my ex-husband, George, was killed instantly in a freak automobile accident. Although we had been divorced for almost fifteen years, we shared two grown daughters and since George and his new family still lived in Fairfax, we remained friendly. Needless to say, I was very upset at his untimely death. A call that I responded to only a week later helped me deal with it.

I was at home, watching TV. "Fairfax Police to the ambulance corps," I heard over my radio.

"Ambulance on."

"The ambulance is needed for a serious head-on collision on Route 10 across from the Methodist Church." Right down the road from my condo, I thought. "There are reported to be at least two serious injuries."

"10–4. 45–01 will be responding. Tone out for a crew

for a second rig and have it respond." There was a pause. "And you better put the helicopter on standby."

By the time the transmission ended I was on the phone to the police, telling them that I would go directly to the scene. I hadn't taken a call since my ex-husband's death, but I knew I needed to get back to doing the things that were important to me.

I jumped in my car, drove the short distance to the scene of the accident, and arrived just after the first ambulance. As I pulled my car off the roadway I saw the remains of two cars. A large, dark-blue, late-model pickup truck lay in the middle of the road, and a Nissan Stanza stood on its side resting against a tree. From a quick assessment of the cars I gathered that the two vehicles had met, head on, driver's front to driver's front. The front-end damage to each vehicle was extensive; the length of each hood had been reduced by half. Both windshields were demolished.

At the scene of an auto accident, we try to look over the damage to the cars. The "mechanism of injury" is a good indication of the possible damage to the occupants. This accident had probably caused serious injury to both drivers.

The only victim I could see was someone lying in the middle of the road, almost completely surrounded by firefighters and two white-shirted members of the ambulance crew. Both EMTs were working furiously on the injured person.

As I ran up I saw Fred Stevens cutting up the jeans legs of the injured person while Pam Kovacs set up oxygen and controlled the patient's airway. "What can I do?"

Fred looked startled to see me. "Are you all right with this?" he asked me. Since there had been considerable newspaper coverage of my ex-husband's accident a week earlier, people at the corps knew about my loss. "It's bad, Joan."

"I'm okay. What do you need?"

"According to Tim, the man in the other car is DOA. Can you double-check for me? Are you okay with that?"

"Will do." Tim Babbett, now beside the rig assembling a collar and a longboard, was not yet an EMT, and I could understand Fred's desire to reconfirm his findings. In this, a triage situation, the shortage of personnel would dictate the type of care we could give to each victim.

Ordinarily we do CPR if a victim has no vital signs and is not "obviously dead." Our protocol strictly defines obvious death. Rigor mortis, the stiffening of a body after death, and dependant lividity, the pooling of the blood in the lowest parts of the body, are two of the criteria. Decapitation or severe charring are other reasons for not starting CPR. In the absence of these factors, ordinarily we "work the code."

In a triage situation, however, one in which there aren't enough trained people to do what's necessary, we use our skills on the patient who can be saved. In this case, with only the four of us, it would be difficult, if not impossible, to do CPR on one driver, who probably hadn't a chance anyway, and properly care for the other man, a person who could be helped. If the driver of the Nissan had a pulse, however, we'd have to split the crew and work on both patients as best we could.

Part of me didn't want to examine a dead body, particularly at this time, but it had to be done.

I walked over to the Stanza, which was lying at a crazy angle on its side, and saw the driver draped against the door, his head and face covered with blood. I pulled on a pair of gloves, wriggled into the passenger compartment, and reached for the man's carotid pulse. Nothing. I could see brain material through an open wound on the top of the man's head, and it didn't take advanced training to detect obvious, fatal head injuries.

I glanced down and saw what I had suspected. No seat belt.

On television, victims often recover from devastating head injuries like the one I had just seen. In the real world, miracle recoveries are just that, miracles. Unless God intervenes or the patient is very, very lucky, head injuries like this one are fatal.

I slid back out, shook my head at the cops standing beside the car, and trotted back to Fred. "No chance," I said, pulling off my bloody gloves. I looked down at the seriously injured man, now lying seminaked on the ground. Here was a person I could help, someone for whom I could make a difference.

As I pulled on a fresh set of gloves, the man began to thrash around, his bloody arms trying to push the two EMTs away. He succeeded in removing the oxygen mask that was probably his best chance for improvement. Fred was trying to bandage the man's sucking chest injury, and Pam was attempting to take the man's blood pressure.

"Joan," Fred said to me, "take his head and do your best to calm him down and keep the oxygen on him. Talk to him and hold his head tightly. We've got the chopper coming, a five-minute ETA."

I took the man's head between my palms and pressed tightly. "Sir," I yelled into his ear, "we need you to stay still. We're trying to help you but you have to hold still." His breathing was shallow and very rapid, too fast to be doing him much good. He needed to be ventilated, but there was no way we could do that until he was a lot calmer.

While I tried to control the man's head, Tim put a cervical collar around his neck and fastened the Velcro closure. I adjusted the oxygen mask so it again fitted closely to his face. "Sir, try to breathe easy. The oxygen will help you." I looked up. "Do we know his name?"

"Mitch," Fred said. He looked over at the crowd

gathered beside the road and pointed to a man in a denim jacket. "He was a passenger in this guy's truck. He's got a broken arm but he can wait."

"Mitch," I yelled into his ear, "try to calm down and breathe more slowly. We're taking good care of you and the helicopter is on the way." The man's movements calmed and I could feel him try to slow his breathing. "That's better," I said. "Try to relax and let us take care of you."

"Chest trauma," Fred said, "with a few broken ribs. I bandaged the sucking wound and I heard diminished sounds on the left side. Serious pneumo- possibly hemo-thorax." The man's chest was in bad shape. He had an opening through the chest wall. Air and possibly blood had entered his chest cavity, a life-threatening condition.

Fred had placed a tight plastic bandage over the hole, leaving one corner free as a flutter valve so air could escape but not reenter the chest. Despite all our best efforts, however, the injury was restricting Mitch's ability to get air into his lungs. Hypoxia, lack of oxygen, was affecting his level of consciousness and causing his combative behavior.

"Oxygen seems to be helping," I said. "His color is improving but we still may need to bag him." I leaned down and spoke into Mitch's ear. "You're doing much better. Breathe slowly and deeply. In and out, in and out." His breathing improved a bit. "Rate's about 28," I said.

"Respirations of 28 ought to be able to support him for the moment," Fred said. "Just watch his head and monitor his airway."

"Will do."

"He also has bilateral, closed femur fractures," Fred said. "Tim, get the MAST. We'll use them to immobilize the legs." Shit, I thought. Both thigh bones were broken, although the bone ends hadn't punctured the skin.

Pam finished taking vitals. "Pulse 120 and weak, respirations 28 and shallow, BP 90 over 65." She covered the man's upper body with a blanket to preserve his body heat.

Tom brought the military antishock trousers and quickly assembled them. Like a full, lower-body blood-pressure cuff, the MAST, when inflated, would both immobilize the man's legs and help to treat his shock.

While I held Mitch's head, the rest of the crew slipped the MAST on and got a long backboard under him. Pam took another set of vitals. This time Mitch's blood pressure had dropped to 85 over 65. "Let's inflate," Fred said. They quickly used the footpump to inflate the legs and abdominal compartments of the MAST.

At the first pulsing roar of the helicopter, we all instinctively crouched over the patient to protect him from the tornado of leaves, dirt, and debris that filled the air as the "bird" landed. Two flight nurses ran over and quickly started IV lines in both of Mitch's arms. We hustled him into the back of the chopper and, with less than five minutes total on-the-ground time, the helicopter took off, leaving us to watch its ascent.

"Nice job, guys," Fred said. "We did good."

I sighed as the helicopter gained altitude. "Yeah, we did." I had made a difference, and I felt good for the first time in a week. While Fred, Pam, and Tim cared for the passenger with the broken arm, I caught my breath, then returned home.

I read in the paper that Mitch had been admitted to St. Luke's Trauma Center in critical but stable condition and the passenger had been treated and released. By the time the reporter wrote the story, three days after the accident, Mitch's condition had improved.

And I had made a difference.

In a town like Fairfax, with five elementary schools, all named for presidents, a large middle school, and an equally large high school, we can count on at least one sports-related injury a week during baseball, football, basketball, and soccer seasons.

Most of our younger patients are wonderful in a crisis. They try their best to be strong and cooperative, especially when the other members of their team are watching. I remember an eleven-year-old boy I picked up at a middle-school baseball game.

We arrived in back of Fairfax Middle School and approached a group of uniformed players standing around a boy in full catcher's "body armor" lying in the dirt at home plate. Another group of players stood nearby, all dressed in the Fairfax navy and white. "What happened?" I asked no one in particular. I assumed that anyone who had some information would answer.

"He got hit," one boy said.

"Don't tell," another muttered. "He'll get in trouble."

"We gotta tell. She's a paramedic."

"I'm an EMT and I don't know what trouble he'd get into but I've got to know what happened."

"Nothing," the injured boy answered, trying to stand up. I knelt and put my hands on the boy's shoulders to keep him from standing up before I knew what was going on.

"I'm fine," the boy continued. He looked at one of the other boys. "Did we win?" His voice was steady, but his hands shook.

"We will," said a redheaded boy with his cap and a baseball mitt in his hands. "We're in the fifth inning and we're leading seven to two. But don't worry about the score. You just get well." He snuffled, trying not to let any of his teammates see how upset he was.

I turned to one of the men standing around the supine boy. "Can any of you tell me what happened?"

"He was warming up our relief pitcher without his mask."

Another man chimed in. "Robby's got one hell of a fastball." He motioned toward the redhead then turned back to my patient. "I'm afraid that Chuck got it right in the face."

I looked over the boy's face carefully. There was a round, bright-red mark in the exact center of his forehead and the area was starting to swell. I gently palpated the area of the injury and found no sign of depressed skull fracture. But that didn't mean that there was no serious head injury.

"You'd better take head stabilization," I said to Tom Franks. Any head trauma violent enough to cause an injury that obvious might have done serious head and neck damage. "You're lucky," I said to the boy on the ground. "The ball didn't hit you in the nose or mouth, and there seems to be no cosmetic damage. You'll be just as gorgeous as before you got hit." While Tom took the boy's head between his palms, I asked Fred Stevens to get the collar bag and a longboard. "Your name's Chuck?" I asked.

"Yes, ma'am," he answered.

"Do you remember getting hit?"

"Hit with what?" he asked.

"I gather you got hit in the face with a baseball."

"I did?" He looked at one of the other players.

"It wasn't my fault," Robby said. "I didn't mean to hit you."

"I'm sure Chuck knows that," I said.

"Did we win?" Chuck asked again.

"It's the fifth inning, Chuck," Robby said. "But we're winning seven–two."

Although his speech was clear and not slurred, I wasn't happy about his level of consciousness. He wasn't "all there."

"Okay, Chuck," I said, "we're going to take you over to the hospital and let them examine you." I looked around. "Does someone have parental consent so we can get him taken care of at the hospital?"

"I have," one of the men said. "I'll go with him. I'm the coach."

"Can someone notify his parents?"

"We're from Miller's Pond," the coach said. "It took us almost two hours to get here by bus. I hate to worry his folks when they're so far away."

"His parents will need to talk to the emergency room doctor so they can discuss whatever treatment is necessary. Maybe you can call them from the hospital." Fred returned with the collar bag and board. "Chuck," I said, getting the boy's attention, "we're going to put a collar on you to remind you not to move your head."

"Okay." He looked at Robby. "Did we win?"

"We're winning," one of the boys answered impatiently.

"Why does he keep doing that?" Robby asked.

"He got his bell rung," Fred answered. "I used to play football and this kind of thing happened to me several times."

"Is he okay?" Robby asked.

"I think he's going to be fine," Fred answered. "And we'll get him checked out at the hospital just to be sure."

We finished putting a rigid cervical collar around his neck, then carefully rolled Chuck onto the longboard. As we lifted him, he asked again, "Did we win?"

"Why does he keep asking the same question over and over?" the coach asked.

"He is having trouble with short-term memory," I answered. "He's concerned about the game and so he asks about the score. The problem is that he doesn't remember the answer or even that he already asked the question, so he asks again a few minutes later."

"Are you sure he's going to be okay?"

"Let's get him to Fairfax Hospital and they'll examine him, maybe do an X ray." We put Chuck, on the backboard, onto the stretcher and lifted him into the rig.

On the way to the hospital, he asked about the game several more times.

We were delayed at the hospital so that by the time we left they had finished taking X rays of Chuck's head and neck. They had discovered that, although he had a concussion and they were going to keep him overnight for observation, there was no indication of serious injury. I found out later that Chuck's team had, indeed, won.

Some of our young patients are very difficult to deal with.

We had been called to the field behind the middle school for a soccer injury. When we arrived, we found a thirteen-year-old girl, lying on the ground, surrounded by a group of other girls.

"What happened?" I asked.

"She fell, twisted her knee, and then I fell over her," a young girl with long brown braids answered, sniffling. "I must have kicked her because she didn't move for a long time." The girl had clean marks made by rivulets of tears down her filthy cheeks.

I bent down and spoke to the groggy girl, lying in the dirt. "Hi, my name's Joan. What's yours?"

"Shelly," she said.

"Well, Shelly, how do you feel?"

"My knee is killing me. And the side of my head hurts behind my ear where Trish kicked me." She closed her eyes and seemed to drift off.

"Okay," I said, treating her as if she could hear everything I said, "let me have a look at you."

I palpated her entire body and looked for deformities. Her knee was slightly swollen and a bit discolored, but other than that, she seemed to be fine. For a second time I palpated her entire face and skull and the back of her neck. There was no indication of any head or neck injury.

"Your head seems to be okay," I said, but her eyes remained closed.

"Will she be all right?" the girl with the braids asked. "She's my best friend and I'm really sorry I hurt her."

"I'm sure you didn't mean to fall over her," I answered.

"But she kicked me in the head," Shelly said, suddenly part of the conversation.

"Shelly, I'm sure she didn't mean it. And you seem to be okay."

"But I'm not. I have this sharp pain on the top of my head and my neck hurts." When I first asked her about her injuries, she had referred to the pain as behind her ear; now it was on the top of her head.

Trish walked away and leaned on another girl's shoulder, sobbing.

"Shelly," I said, "are you sure about where she kicked you?"

"I don't want to talk now." She closed her eyes again.

"But, Shelly, Trish seems to be very worried about you." I looked over at the sobbing girl. "Maybe before you go to the hospital, you should tell her you'll be okay."

Slowly Shelly's eyes opened. "Maybe I won't be. She kicked me real hard." I was becoming very angry. This young snip was milking the situation for all it was worth. I vowed that it wasn't going to affect my treatment, although all I wanted to do at that moment was give Shelly a good spanking.

Nick Abrams walked up with the collar bag, Stephanie DiMartino close behind. "Why don't you put her in a collar," I suggested, "and then we can board her." I paused, then looked at Trish. "I want to talk to her friend for a moment." I walked up to the girl, her braids bobbing up and down as she sobbed. "Trish," I said, placing my hand on her shoulder. I couldn't say too much but I wanted to reassure her. "Don't worry, Trish. I'm sure that Shelly will be fine. And she knows that you didn't kick her on purpose."

"Are you sure she'll be okay?"

I smiled. "I can almost guarantee it."

Trish walked over to her "friend." "Oh, Shelly, she says you'll be okay. Isn't that great?"

"I don't know how she can say that," Shelly snapped. "She doesn't know." Nick had finished fastening the cervical collar around her neck and was positioning the longboard so we could logroll her onto it. "I'm cold," she whined.

"We'll get you a blanket when we get you onto the stretcher," Nick answered.

"But I'm cold now."

Trish unzipped her Fairfax sweatshirt-jacket and held it out. "You can borrow my jacket," she said. We rolled Shelly onto the board. "Here," Trish continued, "I'll put it over you." She draped the jacket over her friend. I could see the soccer-ball logo and the words FAIRFAX GIRLS' SOCCER embroidered on the back.

When Shelly said nothing, I said, "Thank you, Trish. I'm sure that will help a lot." Together Nick, Stephanie, and I strapped Shelly to the longboard and then to the stretcher.

I try to treat all of my patients alike, but Shelly made charm difficult. I positioned myself in the crew seat behind her head and let Stephanie do most of the talking on the way to the hospital. I never found out whether her knee was more than just twisted, but I never doubted that her head injury was nonexistent.

During the roller-skating craze of the early 1980s, some enterprising soul converted an out-of-business supermarket into a roller rink. Each Saturday we'd get a call or two. I particularly remember the evening when the powers-that-be at the rink wouldn't stop the skating for us to immobilize the victim of a potentially serious fall. We put a collar on a delightful eleven-year-old girl and then logrolled her onto a longboard with skaters veering left and right and heavy rock music blaring.

There were two unusual calls at the local golf course one spring a few years ago, within days of each other.

Al Stark had been a golfer even before his doctor advised him to do some gentle exercise to help his borderline high blood pressure. After this advice, Al played eighteen holes whenever possible, keeping his clubs in his partner's cart and walking the entire course. He had to admit that he hadn't ever felt better.

One Saturday morning, Al had a mildly upset stomach as a result of ongoing constipation, but he decided to play anyway. He and his friend Frank McDonald had reached the fourteenth fairway when Al realized that he finally had to move his bowels. Immediately. Embarrassed, but with no time to make it back to the clubhouse, he deliberately sliced his next shot into the woods and disappeared after his ball. When he was sure he was out of sight, he dropped his pants to let nature take its course. As he strained to finish, he felt dizzy and weak. Suddenly his vision began to tunnel, he started to sweat, and, struggling to pull up his pants before he fainted, he collapsed.

"Al," Frank called a few minutes later. "Where did you disappear to? Al? Answer me!" Walking into the woods after his friend, Frank almost stumbled over Al's body. "Al," he called, leaning down and banging his friend's shoulder. "Are you okay?"

Al groaned, slowly swimming up from the blackness.

Frightened for his friend's safety and knowing about his high blood pressure, Frank yelled for help.

A woman in red slacks, a white polo shirt, and golf shoes came crashing through the underbrush. She saw Al's body and cried, "What happened?"

"My friend collapsed. I'm afraid he's having a heart attack."

"I've got a phone in my cart," the woman said, running back toward the fairway.

"Don't move," Frank told Al. "We'll have some help here very soon."

Groggy, Al tried to gather his thoughts as Frank talked incessantly, attempting to ease his own fears.

The ambulance and duty crew had been called to a home where a woman was having chest pains. Fifteen minutes later, a second-rig call had come in for a 10–3, unknown medical emergency, at the golf course. I drove to headquarters and met Sam Middleton and Jill Tremonte. It was agreed that I'd be crew chief.

We responded quickly and were able to drive the ambulance down a fire path quite near where Al still lay in the undergrowth. He was pale, sweaty, and shaking. As we approached, he tried to stand. "I'm feeling better now," he said.

"What happened?" I asked.

"I felt faint and just blacked out. It's nothing."

"It's not nothing," I said. "You fainted and we should find out why."

"Just give me a minute to rest and I'll be fine."

To remember to ask all the necessary questions at the scene of a medical emergency, we use the acronym SAMPLE. Symptoms and general condition of the patient, allergies, medications, past medical history, last meal, events leading up to the incident. I started at the beginning.

"What's your name?"

"My name's Al. Al Stark."

"Okay, Al. My name's Joan. Does anything hurt?"

He hesitated. "No, not really. I'm just a bit shaky."

Maybe this is a bee sting or spider bite, I thought. "Are you allergic to anything?"

"Not that I know of."

"Do you take any medications on a regular basis?"

"No."

If he was so healthy, why had he passed out? I wondered. I continued my information gathering. "Any medical history I should know about?"

"I have high blood pressure, but I don't take any medicine."

"Has anything like this ever happened before?"

"No," Al answered.

"What were you doing when this happened? Or right before?"

"Well," the man hesitated, "that's a little hard to answer." He gazed at his friend.

"I didn't see it," Frank said, trying to help. "He just sliced his ball into the rough and disappeared. I found him just like this."

"Okay, Al. Do you have any idea why this happened? Did this happen suddenly?"

"Well ..." His voice dropped to almost a whisper. "Can I tell *him*?" He pointed to Sam Middleton.

A guy thing, I guessed, but I'd settle for anything. "Sure."

I backed away as Sam leaned over and the two men conversed in whispers. Then Sam sat back on his heels and valiantly tried to stifle his laughter. He quickly took a set of vitals. "As I suspected, his pressure is a bit high, about 160 over 100. I think Al will be fine, but let's transport him anyway so that the hospital can look him over thoroughly."

With Sam taking over as crew chief, we transported Al to Fairfax General. When we were finally back in the rig, I asked Sam what the story was. "Did he ask you not to tell?"

"Nah, it was just real personal."

"So?" I asked.

"He was taking a dump in the woods," Sam said, a

big smile on his face. "The straining probably spiked his blood pressure and he fainted."

"Can that happen?" Jill asked.

"Sure," Sam said. "Taking a shit, especially if you're pushing real hard, often raises the BP. A vasovagal reaction, I think it's called. It's usually minor, but in this case, very embarrassing." He paused. "He was scared shitless, so to speak."

"Oh, Sam." I groaned.

"No shit," Sam continued. "I guess you could say he had a shitty day." He roared at this own humor.

For weeks, Sam's usual foul language was spiced with many more "shits" than ever. His favorite question to anyone who would listen was "Do bears shit in the woods? No, but golfers do."

About a week later, I was hanging around at headquarters, visiting with my daughter Judy, who was a member of the corps at that time and on duty for the afternoon. The call came in for a lawn mower accident at almost the same location on the golf course. Judy was crew chief, Linda Potemski drove, and I went along as the attendant. When we arrived on location, we found a man lying in some longish grass, completely naked. Nearby we saw an overturned, riding lawn mower. The area stank of gasoline.

"What happened?" Judy asked, unfazed by the man's nudity.

At first the man tried to use his hands to cover his genitals, but seeing Judy's lack of interest in his body except where he might be injured, he dropped them. "Get some water and wash me down. Quick. It's burning me."

"We were afraid to do anything," a bystander said.

"What happened?" Judy asked the naked man.

"The mower overturned on me. I got it off, but I was covered with gasoline. Especially in my . . . lap. I stripped my clothes, but I got dizzy from the fumes. Wash me off. The gasoline is still burning me."

"Get me several bottles of sterile water," Judy yelled, stabilizing the man's head. "And we'll have to immobilize him, just in case." I ran toward the rig and looked for the water. Poor man, I thought. Just his luck that we were an all-female crew. Although we know there's no sex in first aid, it's hard to convince our patients.

"How's your head, neck?" Judy asked. "Any injuries?"

"No. I'm fine, except for the gasoline."

While Linda got the longboard and collars, I found three 1000 cc containers of sterile saline. I've always wondered why we have these, I thought. Now I know. Just in case. I also grabbed the plastic sheet we use in the rain, a blanket, and several small towels. When I arrived back beside Judy, I dropped the rest of the items and twisted off one of the bottle caps.

"Any gasoline on your face or in your eyes?" Judy was asking, grabbing the plastic sheet and using it to shield the man from the eyes of bystanders.

"No, just my . . . uh . . . thighs and such."

It was the "and such" that was causing the problem.

"Okay, Mom, pour away," Judy said. I sloshed the entire bottle of water over the man's genitals and opened a second.

"That's your mom?" the man asked.

"Yeah. We do this together sometimes," Judy said as she handed him a towel. He patted himself down, not meeting anyone's eyes.

"That's great," he said as I poured the second bottle of water over his body.

"Better?" I asked.

"Much," he answered, heaving a sigh.

We poured the third bottle over him and, when he had dried himself off, we covered him with a blanket. His vital signs were good so we quickly immobilized him and transported him to Fairfax Hospital, where he was treated for his gasoline burns, then released. Judy and I still talk about that call.

Short Subjects

Ed and I are glad when a potentially bad situation isn't as serious as the dispatch information had made it seem.

The police phoned us one night.

"The alarm has gone off in the toxic gas room at Monroe Plastic Products," the dispatcher told me.

MPP was a research and manufacturing facility located at one end of town. We knew from informational sessions we had had in conjunction with the fire department that no one, including the scientists who worked there, was sure exactly what the storage rooms contained.

"The fire department's responding," I was told, "and they've alerted the county haz-mat team." I hoped that the hazardous materials experts would have nothing to do. I hoped that *we* would have nothing to do. "The fire department wants you, just in case." I hung up the phone and Ed and I began to dress.

As I relayed the story to Ed, he muttered, "In case of what? And what the hell do we know about decontamination?"

"No clue," I said.

As we sped south, down the parkway, I looked at Ed and said, "Sometimes I wonder why we do these things. Why are we going this way? If the danger is south, I want to go north." We continued south.

We waited in the parking lot for three hours while experts gathered and tests were run. Fortunately, the alarm had sounded in error.

What we would have done if there had been a real

toxic gas leak, I still don't know. They've cleaned out that facility since our call. Thank heavens.

The tones went off at headquarters. "A full crew is needed at Upland Meats for a man with his hand caught in a grinder." I was on duty so I responded with the crew, albeit reluctantly. When we arrived at the scene, we found Marcus DeMill with his hand caught deep in his meat grinder. "I'm really okay," he said. "One finger's caught and crushed but I don't think I'm bleeding at all."

"How did this happen?"

"Don't ask. I've been in this business for seventeen years, and this has happened maybe three times before."

"How are we going to get you out?" I asked.

"Mark, my son, is coming. He knows how to take this thing apart."

Three burly firemen rushed in, ready to dismantle the machine with axes and the Hurst Tool. "Not a chance," Marcus yelled. "If I can wait, you can."

We waited until Mark arrived, and the firemen helped him take the grinder apart. As Marcus had known, only his index finger was injured. We splinted it and drove him to the hospital. He was fine. Thank heavens.

"The ambulance is needed for a child who's swallowed half a bottle of peroxide." Damn, I thought, climbing into the driver's seat of the rig. I turned to Pam Kovacs, who was riding in the passenger seat. "Why don't you call the police and have the officer at the scene call poison control. Let him find out what they have to say."

"Good idea," Pam said, and radioed Fairfax police.

Hoping that we could get there in time, I raced through town. "Fairfax Police to the ambulance responding to the call for the child who swallowed peroxide."

"45–01 on," Pam said.

"Poison control says that peroxide isn't poisonous. You can respond with caution just to calm the parents down."

"10–4," Pam said, replacing the mike in its holder. "Did you know that peroxide isn't poisonous?"

"Nope, but I do now." Thank heavens.

Chapter 4

"Roy," Adelaide Herrington called. "Roy, I need my morning medications, dear." Seventy-six-year-old Adelaide Herrington had been bedridden for more than five years. Initially it had been a serious problem for her daughter Grace, but finally she had found a delightful older woman who was thrilled to make some money staying with Adelaide during the day while Grace worked in the city.

Now, since Roy, Grace's twenty-two-year-old son, was between jobs, she had enlisted his help. She had let her regular sitter take a few weeks off and Roy had moved in. He was a caring and, in general, dependable young man, despite a previous drug problem. Grace had been a little concerned about leaving her mother alone with him, but Roy had assured her that he was now clean. And Grace had seen no indication of drug use for many months.

Before Grace had left for work that morning, she had awakened her son and had told Adelaide that Roy would bring her pills and breakfast in a few minutes. Now it had been half an hour since Grace's departure and Adelaide had not seen her grandson, her pills, or breakfast.

"Roy, dear," Adelaide called, more loudly. "Don't forget my medicine. And I'm really getting a bit hungry." She still got no response. Confused by Roy's silence, she waited a few minutes and called again. Frustrated by her inability to get an answer from her grandson, she took the phone from her bedside table and dialed her daughter's car phone.

"Grace dear, it's Mother."

"What's wrong, Mom?" Grace asked, weaving through traffic on her way to the city.

"I can't get any answer from Roy and I haven't had my medications or my breakfast."

"That's odd," Grace said. "He said he would be out of bed in just a minute. Hang up and I'll call back. Don't you answer for a few rings and let him pick up."

Adelaide hung up and almost immediately the phone rang. She let it ring four or five times, then picked up. "Grace?"

"I'm worried, Mom. Now that I think about it, he really didn't look well this morning. I'm going to head home. You call the police."

Adelaide heard her daughter hang up, pressed the redial button, and dialed 911.

I had just gotten into some serious writing and was well into a story for the next book that Joan and I had contracted to write when my Prescott Rescue Squad beeper went off.

"GVK–861 Prescott to the rescue squad. A full crew is needed for an unknown medical at 340 North Highview. Please call in."

I was loath to break my concentration in the middle of my story. It would take me half an hour just to get back into it. But it was 8:00 A.M. Although I was new to Prescott, I had quickly learned their pattern of response, and this hour on weekday mornings was the worst. Of course, the medic would head to the scene immediately, but I knew that there would be few if any Prescott EMTs available.

I punched the speed-dial button on my phone.

"Prescott Fire Department, Rizzo speaking."

"Hi, Andy. It's Ed Herman. I'll respond directly to the scene. It's only a few blocks from my house."

"Okay, Ed. The medic's on the other side of town so he'll be a bit delayed."

A Prescott patrol car was already at the house when I arrived. I could see Officer Mike Gold banging on the door.

"It's locked," he told me as I approached. "I'll go down and try the basement door."

I continued to bang on the front door while Mike did the same downstairs. There was no response. Jack Johnson, another squad member, came up with his personal crash kit and the oxygen he had gotten from the trunk of Mike's police car.

Mike came back to the front door where Jack and I were waiting. "We'll have to make a forceful entry," he said, and, with one strong blow of his foot, kicked the door open.

We could see the boy as soon as we entered the house. He was lying on his back, completely naked. His breathing was agonal, like that of a person who is about to die, certainly not fast enough to sustain life. Without a word, Jack unzipped Mike's oxygen bag and started to hook up the bag valve mask to the oxygen tank. I pulled up the boy's eyelids. The pupils were the size of pinpoints, even in the dim light. I turned toward Mike. "From the looks of him, he's OD'd on narcotics," I told him.

"Yeah, I thought so," Mike replied. "I've arrested him before."

Jack was about to start forcing oxygen into the boy's lungs with the BVM to help him breathe. "Hold it a second, Jack," I said. "I think he's stopped breathing."

I lifted the boy's chin to open his airway, placed my ear near his nose and mouth, and felt for the carotid pulse in his neck. He had a strong pulse but I could hear no breathing. "I've found a pulse. Let's start bagging him." I slipped an oral airway into the boy's throat, tilted his head back, and held the mask against his face. Jack squeezed the bag. We could see the boy's chest rise with each squeeze. We were getting oxygen into his lungs.

Jack and I continued to ventilate the boy artificially as additional rescue squad members arrived. Jack pressed his fingers against the boy's neck. "He's still got a pulse," he said. "What's the ETA on the medic?"

"The medic 'bus' just pulled up," Mike replied. Since I had only recently begun riding with Prescott, I hadn't yet gotten used to the term "bus," which had become an annoying nickname for the fly car just as their head-quarters was known as the "barn."

As we continued artificial ventilation, Paramedic Hugh Washington walked in. "Waddya got, guys?" he asked.

Jack answered, "Probably OD. He's got a good ca-rotid pulse but he's in respiratory arrest. Pupils are pin-point."

"Okay," Hugh said calmly, "keep ventilating him while I start a line and get some Narcan into him."

Hugh began whistling to himself as he slowly and calmly began to assemble his equipment. Jack and I looked at each other and at Hugh. Neither of us had dealt with a narcotics overdose before, but we knew that the only thing keeping this kid alive was our bag-ging him. "Hugh, this kid's in respiratory arrest," I re-peated, thinking that perhaps he had not heard Jack.

"Yeah, yeah, I know. Just keep bagging him. Do it faster. Hyperventilate him until I'm all set up." Jack was starting to get tired from squeezing the bag, so I took over while he held the mask. I squeezed the bag as quickly as it refilled with oxygen from the previous squeeze, about once every two or three seconds instead of the usual one breath every five seconds.

One of the squad members who was standing by asked, "Ed, do you want us to bring up the stretcher or the stairchair?"

There was a steep flight of stairs up to the front door, and it would be difficult to carry the boy down on the stretcher. But I didn't know whether he would be able to sit up in the stairchair. "Waddya think, Hugh?" I asked.

Sally Walsh arrived driving the ambulance. She ran into the house and Hugh handed her an IV bag. "Purge the line for me, Sally," he said softly. While Hugh rummaged in the drug box, Sally efficiently started the flow of fluid and eliminated all of the air from the IV system so that no bubbles would go into the boy's vein.

"Hugh, stretcher or stairchair?" I asked again.

Hugh had stopped whistling. Now he was humming. "Neither one," he answered. "Narco ODs walk to the ambulance."

Again Jack and I looked at each other. The kid we were working on was for all practical purposes dead. I wondered what Hugh had been smoking, as he hummed a tune while inserting a needle into a vein of the boy's arm. Having secured the line with tape, Hugh now reached into his bag, withdrew a vial, and drew up the contents into a hypodermic syringe.

"Okay, guys, I'm going to inject Narcan into the line," Hugh said, his voice matter-of-fact. "You can stop bagging him. And you'd better move back."

"But he's still not breathing," I protested.

"Well, you can stay there if you want to, but some guys get real pissed off at you for ruining a good high. I wouldn't want to be within swinging range of him when I push this Narcan."

Reluctantly Jack and I removed the BVM and backed away as Hugh pushed the plunger of the hypodermic syringe. Almost instantly, the boy started to breathe, and within seconds, his eyes flew open and he started to sit up. "What happened?" he asked.

Within ten minutes, the boy had gotten dressed, and Hugh, whistling again, was leading him as he walked down the steep flight of stairs. As Roy climbed into the waiting ambulance, Grace drove into the driveway and I quickly explained what had happened. Grace slowly shook her head, then went inside to get her mother's medications and breakfast.

Some calls are just strange.

He had been born Norman Ginsburg, but he had changed his name during his stay at an Indian ashram thirty years earlier. Now he was fifty-one years old with long, stringy, brown hair and a more than full black-and-gray beard. His house smelled of incense and the unfamiliar sweet-pungent aroma was not at all unpleasant.

We found him sitting in a living room chair, leaning forward.

"Hi, I'm Ed. What's your name?"

"Rajij." He groaned, obviously in a lot of pain.

"What happened?" I asked.

"My stomach. It hurts so bad." He gasped.

"How long has this been going on?"

"About three days. But it's much worse today."

"Where does it hurt?"

"All over my belly."

"Where did it hurt when it started?"

He straightened out a little and put his hand on the lower right part of his abdomen.

"Down here," he indicated.

"Rajij, I'm going to examine you. Is that okay?"

"No, no," he protested. "I just called because I need help to brew the herbs I need to cure me. I don't believe in traditional medicine. But I can't walk. If you would just help me with my herbs, I'll be fine."

"Look, Rajij, we're supposed to check you out physically. We'll get into a lot of trouble if we don't do our job. How about letting us examine you first and see what we find, then we can talk about your natural, non-traditional approach to the problem."

The "we will get into trouble if we don't do our job" usually works with recalcitrant patients. Most people don't want you to have problems after you have been nice enough to respond to their call for help.

"Okay," Rajij replied, "but hurry up. Once I get those herbs brewed, I'm sure I'll be better."

I wondered whether he was planning to drink the brew or put it on his abdomen, but decided that I didn't really want to know.

I began to examine Rajij while my other crew members took a set of vitals and got other information from him that we would need. When I touched his abdomen, he screamed and violently pushed my hand away. But he had not removed my hand before I had learned what I needed to know. His abdomen was rigid as a board, an indication of bleeding or infection in his abdominal cavity.

Rajij was probably suffering from a ruptured appendix. He was in big trouble, and time was becoming more and more important. His vital signs—rapid heart rate, rapid respirations, and flushed, hot skin—also indicated a massive infection.

"Rajij," I said calmly, not wanting to alarm him, "I think we should take you over to the hospital and let the doctors look at you."

"Definitely not," he answered. "My herbs and meditation will heal me."

I decided that I did not have time to waste on a discussion of the merits of traditional versus holistic medicine. Many physiological problems can be treated successfully by "nontraditional" means. This wasn't one of them.

I hardened my tone of voice. "Okay, Rajij. I don't like to scare my patients, but we really don't have time to fool around. I don't know exactly what's wrong with you, but I know enough to be sure that if we don't get you to the hospital stat, you may very well die. Do you know what stat means? It's a medical term that means 'as fast as we can haul our asses.' "

He stared at me so I continued. "We can't force you

to go to the hospital. If you refuse our help, I'll ask you to sign a release saying that we offered to treat you and take you to the hospital, but that you refused. I'll have it witnessed by the police officer, and we'll leave. My guess is that we will have to come back later today, but by then it will probably be too late to save you."

I hated to use this approach, but I was being very honest. I believed every word that I said to Rajij. This kind of hard, direct approach didn't always work, but I didn't know how else to get him to go to the hospital fast.

Rajij looked at me and I could see the uncertainty in his eyes. "You need this. Now," I said. When he nodded his head slightly, I knew that I had been successful. We brought the stretcher over, next to his chair.

"Can you stand up and swing your butt onto the stretcher?" I asked.

Rajij tried to stand but fell back into the chair. "No. It hurts too much," he said. "I can't walk at all."

"How long have you been in this chair?" I asked.

"Oh, I came down from upstairs right after I called you guys."

I was completely puzzled. He couldn't stand up, but he had walked down a flight of stairs twenty minutes earlier?

"How did you get down the stairs?" I asked.

"I meditated down the stairs, man. I meditated down the stairs."

Within a few minutes, we had lifted Rajij up and gotten him onto the stretcher, sitting up, with pillows under his knees to keep them flexed, and were on the way to the hospital—code 3.

Twenty minutes later, as my crew and I were leaving the emergency room, we paused to look back. We glimpsed one of the strangest sights we had ever seen in our emergency medical careers. Rajij had somehow gotten himself into the leg-twisted, full-lotus position on the gurney and was chanting while the ER physician and three nurses pleaded with him to allow them to treat him. The last thing I could hear as we wheeled our stretcher out of the ER was Rajij chanting "Nam-yoho-orengay-kyo, nam-yoho-orengay-kyo . . ."

In layperson CPR classes, students are taught to deal with cardiac arrest due to a heart attack or choking. These are the situations in which CPR is most likely to save a life. But a heart also may stop functioning as a result of serious injury. Victims of traumatic cardiac arrest, however, are rarely saved. Whatever injury causes a person's heart to stop beating usually does so much damage that neither CPR nor anything else can save him.

The call came in as a self-inflicted gunshot wound. The young man was still breathing when we arrived at the scene, but he was lying in a large pool of blood and the side of his head was gone. He went into cardiac arrest soon after our arrival, and we did CPR all the way to the hospital. I remember his brain tissue dripping on my shoe as I ventilated with the BVM while Jack McCaffrey did chest compressions. I remember wondering how to get brains off shoes—the kind of disconnected thought that many ETMs tend to have at times of horror and futility. The emergency room physician on staff at the hospital "pronounced" him almost immediately after examining his wound.

Sometimes, however, very rarely, we get lucky.

It was a warm, Indian summer Sunday in mid-October. The leaves in Fairfax were at their peak of color. It was the kind of day when people from the city streamed up the parkway to look for places to fish or hike, or just drive the back roads to see the glorious autumn display.

I would be on duty for another hour and then was

planning to hike up to the top of Redtail Hill. In the meantime, I was lying on the lawn in front of FVAC headquarters, basking in the rays of the sun, which, though still warm, was now much lower in the sky than a few months earlier. The air smelled of decaying and illegally burning leaves, and the slight chill in the air, even in the sun, hinted at the frost that would probably coat the Fairfax lawns the following morning.

Suddenly the klaxon sounded.

"Fairfax Police to Fairfax Ambulance."

"Fairfax Ambulance on," Pam Kovacs answered from inside the FVAC building.

"The ambulance is needed for a pedestrian struck by a car on Lakeside Road, just east of the old railroad trestle. Be advised, it's reported to be a serious injury."

"10–4," Pam said. "45–01 is responding to Lakeside, east of the trestle, for a 10–2, car versus pedestrian."

I sprinted toward the rig as Pam got into the "shot-gun" seat and Phil Ortiz got into the back. I flipped on the bank of switches to activate the siren and the seven different sets of flashing lights, then started toward Lakeside Road.

"Pam," I said, not taking my eyes off the road, "maybe we should put the helicopter on standby."

The helicopter, with its highly trained flight nurses and advanced life support capability, was a countywide service that, at the time of this call, had become available only a few weeks earlier. We were still not used to calling for it and usually didn't do so until we arrived at the scene and were sure it was needed.

This call sounded serious, however, and we had been encouraged to put the helicopter on standby because it required several minutes to warm up before it could be airborne. We could always cancel it if we didn't need it.

"Good idea, Ed," Pam replied, picking up the radio microphone. "45–01 to Fairfax Police."

"Fairfax Police on."

"Have county control put the chopper on standby.

We'll advise if we want it to respond when we get to the scene."

"10–4, 45–01. We'll notify county control."

And a few minutes later: "Fairfax Police to 45–01."

"45–01 on."

"Be advised, the bird has been placed on standby, awaiting further instructions."

Coming around a sharp curve on Lakeside Road, we saw a car with serious rear-end damage and its trunk open parked on the grass at one of the popular local fishing spots. Behind the car, a man lay on his back with his legs propped up on what looked like a crate. Another man was kneeling next to him, looking helpless. Officer Eileen Flynn was walking back toward the curve, setting out flares. I pulled the ambulance as far off the road as possible and strode over to the patient.

The man appeared to be in his early thirties. His eyes were closed and his face was pale and covered with sweat. The legs of his trousers were soaked with blood. I stabilized his head to prevent movement and said, "Hi, my name is Ed." The man did not respond.

"Can you hear me?" I yelled. No reply. I listened for his breathing and checked for a pulse in his neck. His pulse was weak and his breathing seemed labored. "We're going to have to assist his breathing," I said to Pam, who waited with the giant crash bag. "Hook up the oxygen to the BVM."

"Phil," I yelled, "radio the police and tell them to dispatch the chopper." I turned to the man who had been kneeling next to the victim. "Do you know what happened?" I asked.

"Yeah, I saw it all. He was getting his fishing gear out of his trunk. A car came from that way." He pointed down the winding road. "The asshole couldn't hold the curve and smashed this guy into his car. I couldn't believe it. He saw what had happened, backed up, then drove off. I didn't get the license number." He took a breath. "I found this crate in the woods and put his legs up on it so that he wouldn't go into shock."

The man had meant well, and under other circumstances his action would have been appropriate, but I silently wondered how much additional damage had been done to the victim's already crushed legs by lifting them up onto the crate.

"Was he conscious?" I asked.

"Yeah. He passed out just before you got here."

"The chopper is on the way," Phil reported as he sprinted back from the rig, "but we'll have to transport him by ambulance to the intersection at Route 10. That's the nearest possible LZ." I nodded. The helicopter required a landing zone of at least sixty feet in all directions, and Lakeside Road just wasn't wide enough.

While I bagged the patient, Pam took vitals and Phil used his shears to cut away the man's trousers. The crushing injuries to his legs and pelvis were massive. I turned to Phil. "Get the MAST, Phil. He's real shocky and the MAST will also stabilize his legs."

Phil went back to the ambulance for the MAST while Pam and I stopped ventilating to check for spontaneous respiration. The man had stopped breathing. I reached toward his neck for his carotid pulse. "He's in full arrest," I said to Pam. "I'll continue ventilating and you can do chest compressions."

We had been performing CPR for about a minute when the man gave a sigh and began breathing on his own. Pam and I looked at each other, unable to believe that we really had brought someone back from a traumatic arrest. While he might be breathing now, he was in very bad shape and we knew that he probably would not make it to the hospital.

Meanwhile, Sam Middleton and Jack McCaffrey, two other FVAC EMTs, had responded to our scene and had started to help Phil maneuver the MAST onto the patient. I didn't know whether they had "buffed" the call after hearing of its seriousness on their scanners or if they just happened to be driving by. And I didn't care. We needed all the help we could get.

We fastened the Velcro straps of the MAST around our patient's legs and abdomen, collared him, and immobilized him to a backboard. As I continued to assist his breathing with the BVM, I could hear the whirring blades of the helicopter pass overhead, en route to the LZ, about a mile away. We quickly loaded the man into the ambulance. Phil drove while I continued bagging him and Pam pumped up the MAST with her foot. I watched with amazement at the grace and ease with which she used the walls, stretcher bars, and a ceiling rail to keep from being thrown around in the ambulance, which was speeding along the winding road.

At the landing zone, the helicopter flight nurses climbed into the ambulance, quickly got a tube down into the patient's trachea to assure that his airway would remain open, and started an IV. Within minutes, the patient was loaded into the helicopter and the chopper had lifted off and was on its way to St. Luke's trauma center.

As we watched the helicopter disappear into the sky, none of us who were involved with the rescue believed that the man would live. But he did. And the lifesaving award certificate that we received for that call is very special because not many EMTs have been able to save someone who has had a traumatic cardiac arrest.

Sometimes I think that one of the one things that makes EMTs different from people who are not involved in emergency rescue work is our respect for automobile safety devices, especially seat belts and air bags. It amazes me that people who may be afraid of flying, a risk approximately the same as that of being hit by lightning, will put a child into a car without a seat belt and drive off without giving it a thought.

Most people have a false sense of safety in their car. It feels like part of their home. But I know the danger they are in. I know what can happen to them, and I know how they can protect themselves. If they could feel some of the tragedy that I have witnessed. . . .

The image of the dead child lying on the pavement after being thrown out of a car during a minor fender-bender will always be engraved in my mind. It took me a long time to get over that call, and I still feel rage at the mother who so stupidly and senselessly caused her son's death. In contrast, there was a picture in last week's local newspaper of a car so completely demolished that it was difficult to believe that anyone had survived. But the driver had. And I had been there.

The elderly man had been driving north on the parkway at about sixty miles per hour when he had dozed off. His car had veered off into the woods and struck a tree. I didn't expect to find anyone alive when I approached the wreckage, but the driver was awake and conscious, although in terrible pain. His leg had been broken by the engine, which had been pushed into the bottom of the passenger compartment. We had needed to use the jaws of life to get him out.

The extrication had been long, difficult, and extremely painful for the man, but he had suffered no major injuries other than a badly fractured lower leg. If he had not been wearing a seat belt, his chest would have been crushed by the steering wheel, his head would have gone through the windshield, or, if he had been thrown out of the car, his body would have continued to travel at high speed until it was splattered against a tree or broken to pieces on the ground.

It's not just me. All of us who are involved in the horror of automobile accidents, especially when they needn't be as tragic as they are, recognize the danger.

"Mommy, Mommy. I want some ice cream," Jimmy Grey shouted as the car traveled past Carvel.

"Not now dear," his mother, Cathy, said, driving through the heavy, early-evening traffic. "We're going to have dinner as soon as we get home."

"But I want some."

"Maybe after dinner," Cathy said, trying to placate her five-year-old son.

"No, now!" Jimmy shrieked. "I want some now!"

Cathy turned to Jimmy, who was sitting next to her unrestrained. "If you don't stop screaming, I'm going to tell Daddy that you've been a bad boy," she threatened. She didn't realize that the light had changed and that the car in front of her had stopped. Suddenly she felt a thump as she bumped into the car in front of her. Both she and Jimmy lurched forward. Jimmy struck his head against the dashboard.

I had responded with Prescott and the medic. Hugh Washington and I examined the two occupants of the car and were pleasantly surprised. Cathy appeared to be uninjured, and Jimmy had only a minor bump on his forehead and was complaining of slight neck pain.

Just as a precaution, we immobilized the yowling five-year-old with a cervical collar and placed him on a short backboard. "Medic 1 to Prescott Dispatch."

"Go, Medic 1."

"Be advised I'm 10–8, 10–17." Since we didn't need advanced life support, Hugh was back in service, returning to headquarters. "21–01 will be transporting one and a passenger to FGH."

We began our transport of mother and child to Fairfax General, code 2. Jimmy became amazingly cooperative with us once we bribed him with a stuffed rabbit whom he immediately named Oswald. About five minutes from the hospital, I picked up the radio phone. "Prescott 21–01 to Fairfax Emergency."

"This is Fairfax Emergency."

"Be advised we're en route to your location with a five-year-old male victim of a minor PIAA. He appears to be uninjured except for a small area of swelling on his forehead. We have him boarded and collared as a precaution. At 17:14 his BP was 110 over 70, respirations 24, pulse 90 strong and regular, pupils equal and reactive, skin color normal. Our ETA to your location is approximately four minutes."

"Was the child wearing a seat belt?"

"Negative. He bumped his head on the dashboard."

"10–4, 21–01. We'll give you room assignment on arrival."

"21–01 clear."

"Fairfax Emergency clear."

The trip to the hospital was uneventful. To entertain Jimmy, I blew up a latex glove and drew a face on it with a marking pen. Jimmy was delighted with his balloon rooster that had a five-finger cockscomb sticking out of his head.

As the ambulance backed into the emergency room bay, I was surprised to see Kurt Bankcroft, one of the ER nurses, waiting for us. Normally none of the ER staff meets the ambulance unless we request assistance. As I swung the rear doors open, Kurt began to yell. "Let's go. Let's go. Get him in."

I was amazed at Kurt's behavior. Usually he was calm and professional. "He's okay, Kurt," I assured him. "It's only a little bump on his head."

Kurt raised his voice. "Never mind that bullshit. You people always like to play doctor. Just shut up and get him in. Now."

Astounded and angry, my crew and I wheeled Jimmy into the ER and transferred him to a hospital gurney.

A few minutes later, as I was writing up my PCR, the state Prehospital Care Report we fill out for every call, Kurt came over to me. "I'm sorry, Ed," he said. "I was way out of line. But something happened a few nights ago that still has me acting crazy."

Kurt, an auxiliary with the Davenport fire-police, dropped into a chair next to me. "I was working a road-block with the fire-police around a brushfire. We had the road down to one lane so we were guiding traffic around.

"We had the road well flared out but an approaching driver didn't start braking soon enough. I saw the car approaching fast and heard the driver slam the brakes pretty hard. Fortunately, the car avoided hitting anything." I heard Kurt sigh as he remembered that evening.

"The car remained where it was, without moving, while the other cars pulled forward. After a minute or so, the driver pulled up to us and stopped. Her window was open and she screamed, 'My baby, my baby.' I went over to the car, opened the passenger door, and found a three-year-old girl on the front seat unconscious. 'She hit the dashboard when I braked,' the mother shrieked. I examined the little girl and found that she was in cardiac arrest."

Kurt took a shuddering breath. "She had long, curly blond hair, and I noticed her eyes were green as I checked her pupils." His voice shook as he continued. "I did CPR, the ambulance crew worked her, the ER worked her, but it was no use. She was dead. I never found out whether it was a broken neck or a fractured skull or what. I hope you understand. I didn't mean to be rude before, but when I heard that it was an unseat-belted child with a head injury . . ."

"I understand completely, Kurt," I assured him, patting him on the shoulder. "We've all been there ourselves."

"Apologize to your crew for me, will you?" Kurt asked.

"Will do, Kurt. Take care," I replied as I joined my crew and left the emergency room.

This morning, as I was driving through the parking lot of the Mid-County Mall, I saw a car with an out-of-state license plate about to pull out of a parking space. A man was behind the wheel. Next to him sat a woman with a child on her lap. None of them was wearing a seat belt. I had an almost overwhelming urge to pull my car behind them and not allow them to back out until they belted the child.

Instead, I pulled up next to them and said, through the open windows, "Excuse me, sir. I just want to warn you that the local cops will ticket you for not seat-belting your child."

"Maybe you should mind your own business," he said with a snarl as he backed up, then sped away with a squeal of tires.

Feeling somewhat hopeless, I drove home.

As important as our medical skills are, sometimes during serious medical emergencies our ability to inter-act with patients and their families is even more impor-tant. I often feel like an actor, playing the role of a calm, competent doctor-cop-psychotherapist while in-side I feel like an overwhelmed, frightened kid who wants to run away and hide. But there is a lot of satis-faction in knowing that I have successfully fooled ev-eryone and in doing so I have been able to help a patient and his or her family not only medically but also emotionally.

It had taken a lot of persuasion before fourteen-year-old Theresa Presti had been able to convince her parents to allow her to have a pool party.

"I don't know," her mother had said.

"It's a lot of responsibility," her father had declared.

"Just my closest friends," Terry had begged. "Please, please, please."

"Well . . ." Her mother had weakened.

"I guess so," her father had conceded.

The weather cooperated fully. It was ninety degrees in the July sun and, because it had been hot all week, the pool temperature was almost eighty. While ten kids were joyously carrying on in the Prestis' backyard and pool, under the watchful eyes of Mr. and Mrs. Presti, Terry ran into the house to get some more Coke and ice, leaving the sliding door to the deck and backyard open.

As she was pouring ice cubes into a bucket, her mother walked in behind her and slid the door shut. "Theresa, how many times have I asked you to close the door behind you?" her mother said in exasperation. "We can't afford to air-condition the entire outside world."

Between her daydreaming and the sound of the ice cubes, Terry didn't hear her mother's comments. She was too busy thinking about the way the boys were reacting to her new bikini. Her parents hadn't been very happy about her suit either, but, as usual, Terry had gotten her way.

Terry turned, clutching two bottles of Coke and a bucket of ice cubes, kicked the refrigerator door shut, and ran toward the sliding door. She didn't want to miss any of the fun. She had run right through the old nonsafety glass before she realized that the door was closed.

By some miracle Terry was not even scratched by the shattered glass that cascaded down around her. She would not have been injured at all if, in her shock, she hadn't stumbled, fallen backward, and sat on the razor-sharp glass edge that remained at the bottom of the door frame.

I was outdoors, mowing the lawn. My scanner was in my back pocket with a wire leading to an earphone, so I could hear the radio above the roar of the lawn mower in case a call came in. No one was on duty at headquarters, and, on a hot summer weekend day like this, a lot of FVAC and Prescott members were away. There probably weren't many people around to take ambulance calls.

It was a lousy time to be doing heavy work, but with all of the hot, dry weather, the grass had finally stopped growing. If I did one good mowing now, I probably wouldn't have to do it again until September. I can never understand why people fertilize their lawns. Why encourage the stuff to grow? I would rather sprinkle my lawn with a growth retardant so that I don't have to mow it as often. Oh, well, I thought, I guess lush, green lawns are considered desirable.

Suddenly I heard the FVAC pager tones. I leaned forward and pulled back the lawn mower's throttle. The engine sputtered and died.

"Fairfax Police to all FVAC pagers and home monitors. An ambulance is needed at 2130 Sycamore Place for a 10–3, a severe laceration. All units please call in."

Sycamore Place, a cul-de-sac in a housing development, was about two miles away, between my house and FVAC headquarters. I grabbed my FVAC portable radio from my porch and pressed the send key. "45–22 to FPD."

"Go ahead, 45–22."

"I'll respond to the scene. Keep toning out for a driver to pick up the rig and an attendant."

"10–4, 45–22."

As I jumped into my car and turned the ignition key, the pager tones again blared from the radio. "Fairfax Police to all FVAC pagers and home monitors. An attendant and a driver to pick up the rig are still needed for a 10–3 at 2130 Sycamore Place. Please call in."

And about a minute later: "Fairfax Police to 45–22."

I picked up my radio. "Go ahead, FPD."

"45–27 and 45–39 are picking up the rig."

Great, I thought. Marge Talbot and Linda Potemski. I was glad that they were around.

"10–4, FPD. My ETA to location is about 0–2."

"10–4, 45–22."

As I pulled up in front of 2130 Sycamore Place, I grabbed the radio and barked, "45–22 on location," so that the police, Marge, and Linda would know that I had arrived at the scene. Stuffing the radio into my back pocket, I popped the trunk, grabbed my crash kit, and rapidly walked up to the front door.

"Fairfax Ambulance," I shouted as I rang the bell.

The ashen-faced woman who answered the door quickly led me through the kitchen and out to the deck where a group of teenage kids were gathered around a dark-haired girl who lay on her back. She was being comforted by a middle-age, bearded man who was as pale as the woman who had met me. The girl had some large, blood-soaked towels wrapped around her upper left thigh and buttock.

"Hi, I'm Ed. I'm with Fairfax Ambulance." I brushed some glass shards aside and knelt down beside her. "What's your name?"

"Terry Presti," the girl answered.

"I'm her father," the man added, "and that's her mom," nodding toward the woman that had let me in.

I looked up at the group of kids gathered around. "Why don't you kids go down to the pool?" I suggested. "I think Terry needs some privacy." Reluctantly Terry's friends shuffled away.

"What happened?" I asked the girl.

"I ran through the glass door and sat on the broken glass." Her voice was strong and her thoughts were clear.

"It was all my fault," the woman cried. "I closed the door and Theresa didn't realize that it was closed."

I looked up at the distraught woman. "Accidents happen, Mrs. Presti. They're not necessarily anyone's fault."

"But—"

"Are you hurt anywhere else besides your bottom?" I interrupted.

"No," Theresa replied. "But it hurts a lot." She seemed less shaken up than her parents.

I was puzzled by their reaction. The girl appeared to be in good condition, considering what might have happened. "Terry, I'm going to need to examine your cuts. I want you to lie on the side that is not injured. Okay?"

"Sure," she replied, rolling onto her right side.

Usually I wouldn't remove dressings that had already stopped the bleeding. In this case, however, the bunched towels were wet with pool water and not really pressed properly against the wound.

I took some dry, sterile gauze pads from my crash kit, unwrapped them, and then carefully began to remove the blood-soaked towels, expecting to find extensive lacerations. I was totally unprepared for the actual injury. As I slowly removed the bottom towel, Terry's left buttock began to come away with it. I swallowed hard as I saw that one cheek had been almost severed by the edge of the glass. I stared at the exposed globular, fatty tissue. Now I knew why the Prestis were so upset.

I began my acting performance, praying that the trembling of my body would not give me away. I calmly used one hand and my teeth to open the two multitrauma dressings I had in my kit. I held all the pads against the avulsed tissue and pressed her buttock back into its normal position.

"Terry," I said in a voice that I hoped sounded casual and relaxed, "you've got a nasty cut. I'm going to bandage it up and then take you over to the hospital. Okay?"

"I guess so," Terry replied. "Will I need stitches?"

Although I didn't want her to know just how badly she was injured, I never lie to a patient. "Yes, I think so." I answered. "Have you ever had stitches before?" I asked.

"Yeah. I cut my hand while opening a tin can last year and needed four stitches."

"Well, then you know that stitches aren't so bad," I suggested.

"They're not exactly fun," Terry replied.

"No, I guess they aren't," I conceded, "but it certainly does get everyone to be nice to you."

"Yeah," she said, a small smile crossing her face. She glanced at the group of teenagers gathered beside the pool.

By this time the ambulance had arrived, and Marge and Linda had brought up the large trauma kit and the portable oxygen tank from the rig. "Terry, this is Linda and here's Marge. They will be going to the hospital with us."

"Hi, Terry." Marge introduced herself cheerfully, then turned to me. "What do you need, Ed?"

"I'll need about four or five large multitrauma dressings and some roller gauze." I turned to Linda. "Linda, put her on a non-rebreather at twelve liters. She doesn't seem to have lost much blood, but the oxygen can't hurt."

As Marge handed me three more sterile dressings, I placed them so that they completely covered the original dressings and Terry's wound. I held everything in place while Marge used a figure-eight pattern, winding the roller gauze alternately around Terry's thigh and waist to secure the dressings.

Meanwhile, Linda attached a non-rebreather face mask to the oxygen tank, adjusted the valve to a flow rate to twelve liters per minute, held her finger over the inflow valve until the reservoir bag expanded, then gently placed the mask over Terry's mouth and nose. "Just breathe normally," she said to Terry. "The oxygen will help you." Working calmly but quickly, we finished our bandaging, recorded Terry's blood pressure, pulse, and respiration rates, and placed her on the stretcher, lying on her right side.

"Can my mom come with me in the ambulance?" Terry asked as we wheeled the stretcher toward the rig.

Recalling how upset Terry's mother had been, I was reluctant to have her in the back of the rig. But Terry had specifically asked for her, so I decided I'd talk to the woman.

While Marge and Linda settled Tracy in the rig, I

spoke to Mrs. Presti. "We need you to be calm if you're going to ride with her. Can you do that?"

"I think so. It's so bad. Her flesh was just hanging there."

"Let the doctors at the hospital worry about how to fix her up. You just be tough. Yes?"

She took a deep breath. "Yes."

As soon as we got into the rig, I reached into a compartment above the stretcher, pulled out a stuffed bear, and offered it to Terry. "We carry these guys for kids, and I know you're not a kid anymore, but I have a feeling you're not too old for a stuffed animal, are you?"

All the way to the hospital, Terry clutched the teddy bear while her mother sat on the crew bench next to Linda and talked to her daughter. I sat in the crew seat at Terry's head, constantly reassuring her mom with my expression.

When we got into the ambulance to return home, Marge picked up the microphone. "45–01 to Fairfax Police."

"Go ahead, 45–01."

"Be advised we are 10–8, 10–17, returning to base via the scene to drop off 45–22."

"10–4, 45–01."

I looked at my shaking hands and turned to Marge. "Marge, could you do me a big favor?"

"Sure," Marge replied. "What is it?"

"If I go back to headquarters with you, could you give me a lift in your car to Joan's house? This call has me shook up a lot. I'm not sure I'm fit to drive. Joan can drive me back to my car later."

"No problem, Ed," Marge said. "Was the injury that bad? I never actually saw what she had done."

I took a deep breath. "It was one of the largest and deepest lacerations I've ever seen, maybe twelve inches long. Her butt was all but disconnected from her body."

"Wow. I never knew."

Joan and I spent a lot of time talking that afternoon. When I finally got home that evening, I was feeling very grateful that she and I could share experiences.

Although I don't usually contact patients after a call, I stopped by at 2130 Sycamore Place the next day to find out how Terry was doing. Mrs. Presti was looking a lot better than she had when I last saw her. "Theresa is doing fine," she told me. "They took her up to surgery soon after you left. She'll be in the hospital for a few days, but the doctor says she'll be fine." She smiled. "He said he lost count of how many stitches it took."

"I'm glad she's doing well," I said.

"I can't believe how calm you were," she exclaimed. "When I saw how badly she was cut, I almost fell apart. But I guess you are used to things like that. I'm sure you see it all the time, and it probably doesn't bother you."

I smiled, asked her to say hello to Terry for me, and went home thinking that maybe I have missed out on an acting career.

Short Subjects

Sometimes people don't think about what they're carrying in their car.

Joan and I responded to an automobile accident where everyone's injuries were complicated by the load of bricks the driver had been carrying on the backseat. In another, a bowling ball bounced around inside the car, injuring people who might otherwise have walked away from the accident.

Recently our local paper carried a story of a woman who claimed that her auto accident was caused by a helium-filled balloon that her daughter was bringing home from a birthday party. "The damned balloon was bouncing all over the car and suddenly it was in my face. I couldn't see."

A friend of mine arrived at an accident scene and discovered the driver covered with blood. At least she thought it was blood until she found the rest of the raspberries the driver had been picking before the accident.

Although people may always wear clean underwear, "in case they get into an accident," they may not consider the ramifications of the contents of their home.

The fire was spectacular. The entire front of the two-story house was engulfed and sixty-foot-high flames roared into the night sky. Ed and I, both children of the sixties, were quickly able to identify the odd smell that drifted with the smoke. "That's what I think it is, isn't it?" I asked.

Inhaling, Ed said, "It certainly is. I wonder how large a stash the owner had."

It was a cold evening and as the mundane water-pouring work of what is called "surround and drown" extended into the fourth hour, firefighters gathered in their large, heated rescue truck, breathing the marijuana fumes off each other's clothing. It was interesting to watch the parade of police, reporters, and ambulance workers wander into the rescue vehicle to enjoy the aroma pouring from the turn-out gear of those who had been closest to the house.

Chapter 5

The past winter was particularly harsh in Fairfax. As in most of the Northeast, we had record low temperatures and an unusual number of snowfalls.

It was 3 A.M. on a particularly cold Sunday morning in January, and Ed and I were riding our usual midnight-to-6 A.M. shift from my house. We had just returned from a call for a man with difficulty breathing and, as Ed and I turned the knob on the door to my condo, the tones went off again.

"Fairfax Police to the ambulance. Take a mutual aid for Davenport for an unknown medical emergency."

The city of Davenport doesn't have a roster of duty crews the way Fairfax has. In Fairfax, members are required to sign up for duty for at least one shift, or six hours each week. Shifts run from midnight to 6 A.M., 6 A.M. to noon, and so on. Between 6 A.M. and midnight, members on duty ride from headquarters. Between midnight and 6 A.M. members may ride from home, as Ed and I do, as long as they can arrive at headquarters within five minutes of being called.

Usually we have full crews, at least a driver, an EMT, and an attendant, for the evening and midnight shifts. The day shifts are more difficult to fill. In the past there were "housewives" available during the day while their children were at school. Now both men and women work, and few ambulance corps members are available during the daytime hours.

The Davenport Volunteer Ambulance Corps, like the Prescott Rescue Squad, uses a different system to fill ambulance crews. When a call for help comes in, the 911 dispatcher sounds pagers and reports the necessary information. Available members call in and respond. With more than fifty active members, usually the two organizations have little trouble raising crews, days, evenings, or even at 3 A.M.

Occasionally, however, if no one is available or if it has more calls than it can handle, Davenport, like all the neighboring corps, uses the countywide mutual-aid system to summon a nearby squad with its ambulance and crew. On this night, Davenport had called on us for mutual aid.

"Shit," I muttered. "No wonder they can't raise a crew. It's so cold that no one in their right mind would want to go out."

"I guess that means we're not in our right minds," Ed said. "Let's go." He trotted back to his car and climbed into the driver's seat while I got in on the passenger side. As he looked at the temperature gauge on the dashboard, he added, "It's so frigid outside that the car has already started to get cold."

I wanted to know just how miserable I was so, with my teeth chattering, I snapped on the car radio and tuned to our local radio station. "The three A.M. temperature in Fairfax is seven below zero," the announcer intoned.

I sighed. "God, I hate this weather. If I never see another snowflake or feel a temperature below freezing, it will be too soon."

"Seven below, seven above," Ed said. "What's the difference? At three in the morning in the winter it's always cold."

I nodded my agreement.

It was only a few minutes until we pulled into the FVAC headquarters parking lot and ran toward the waiting rig. Even in that brief moment, the blast of cold air was enough to make my exposed face smart. Glad that I had decided to violate the rules and not wear my corps jacket, I snuggled deeper into my down coat.

Bob Fiorella had signed on as a regular for Saturday nights and was waiting behind the wheel of 45–01. "So much for any sleep," he muttered as we pulled out of the lot with me in the front and Ed in the crew seat in the back. "I had just gotten back to bed," Bob complained, thinking of his warm bunk in the crew sleeping quarters. "I was just pulling the blanket up to my nose." He flipped on the flashing lights and drove toward Davenport. "God, I hate when this happens."

Back-to-back calls are unusual, even during the day. Riding midnights, we frequently go for weeks without a call of any kind. Tonight . . .

People don't realize how much stress severe winter cold places on their bodies, and the elderly are especially vulnerable. The seventy-eight-year-old man we had transported on our previous call had been a perfect example. He had walked half a mile to a friend's house earlier in the day and had not felt well after returning home. At about one-thirty in the morning, he had awakened, sweating and panting, with pains in his chest. We had just returned from transporting him to Fairfax General.

"Know where we're going?" I asked Bob. For a change it was easy to hear each other in the front of the rig. Because of the hour and the lack of traffic, we weren't using our siren.

"We've got a Davenport cop car meeting us where Route 10 meets Maple Terrace. He'll lead us in from there. The call's not in a nice area."

Davenport is a small, hundred-year-old city right on the river. Although is has its nicer sections, most of the city is made up of poverty-stricken neighborhoods filled with underemployed families struggling to get by.

This call had been dispatched as an unknown medical, and that told us nothing. It could be anything from a woman in labor to a drug overdose, from a man in cardiac arrest to an abused child.

We followed the Davenport police car down several streets and pulled up behind a second police car, in front of a dilapidated, two-story, wood-frame building. Ed grabbed the crash kit as Bob and I climbed out into the frozen air.

"What's the trouble?" I heard Ed ask the officer who had led us in.

"No real emergency," the officer said. "Call came in to us as a woman with something in her ear."

Did I hear correctly? I wondered. A woman with something in her ear?

We entered the building and walked down a short, dingy hallway into a small bedroom. It was furnished with a wooden dresser covered with flaking white paint and a sagging, overstuffed chair upholstered in what had probably once been a cheerful flowered chintz. On the metal-framed bed a middle-age woman lay curled up on her right side holding her right ear. She was dressed in a heavy sweater, a pair of sweat pants, and heavy socks. She had covered most of her body with a crocheted afghan and a red winter jacket.

As he often does when the patient is a woman, Ed let me take over care. "Hello, ma'am. My name's Joan. What seems to be the trouble?" When she didn't respond, I repeated the question to an unfamiliar officer who was standing, writing on a pad. I saw the small star-of-life pin he wore on his lapel so I assumed he was one of the EMT/police officers recently hired by Davenport. "Officer?" I repeated, when he didn't respond. As I spoke, my breath came out in little white puffs. It was hardly any warmer inside than it had been outside.

"Cockroach in her ear," the officer muttered, totally uninterested. "I took vitals. All within normal range."

"What?" I said, trying not to be shocked. A cockroach in her ear?

"Cockroach in her ear. The right, I think. She wants Fairfax General." He handed me the slip of paper with the patient's name, address, age, vital signs, and pertinent medical information, all efficiently arranged.

I walked up to the woman and asked, "You think something's in your ear?"

"I don't think, I know," she said softly, obviously trying to move as little as possible. "It's a cockroach."

"Which ear?"

"The right one."

"Okay, let's have a look." I pulled out my penlight.

"No light," the officer snapped. "I looked quickly and couldn't see anything obvious. So just take her word for it and go."

Annoyed, I thought, What difference does it make whether I look into her ear or not? I can't do anything about it, whatever it is. I wrapped the woman's coat around her shoulders while Ed and the officer assisted her to a standing position. Crouched and bent over toward her right side, she walked to the stretcher, which we had left outside the front door. We covered her with two blankets and draped a towel over her head to help conserve what little body heat she had.

While en route, I radioed the hospital, saying that we had a patient with a foreign body in her ear. I just couldn't say cockroach over an open radio line. I was sure I'd never hear the end of it back in Fairfax, where many members monitor our radio frequency, even in the middle of the night. And anyway, I wasn't sure I believed it. A cockroach.

When we arrived in the ER, Dr. Margolis was waiting. "Any idea what she's got in her ear?" he asked.

"The EMT officer at the scene said she's got a cockroach in her ear."

Dr. Margolis didn't seem surprised. "Okay. We'll take care of it."

"You mean you believe her?"

He smiled at my obvious naïveté. "It's not unusual in poorer neighborhoods. We've had at least one other in the past week. In this kind of very cold weather, roaches look for a warm place to sleep. Occasionally they crawl into ears just to stay warm."

"I didn't really believe her so I didn't look to see," I confessed.

"It's good you didn't. If you shine a light in, the roach will back up and scratch the eardrum, causing a lot of pain."

"What will you do?"

"We'll take a quick look, then pour in some mineral oil. That will drown the beast and then we can pull him out. It only takes a little while."

I finished my paperwork shaking my head. I guess I am naive. I think I'd like to keep it that way.

Martin Geraldo loved to work in his garden. For seven years, ever since he retired from selling insurance for a huge nationwide company, he had taken most of his spare time and turned the front and back yard of his half-acre home in Fairfax into the showplace of the neighborhood. In the spring, tulips, hyacinths, daffodils, and irises of every color bloomed all around the house.

In the summer, flowers filled the front yard and vegetables took up most of the back. The side yards were planted with blueberry and raspberry bushes, and, as the berries ripened, Martin fought the birds for the harvest. In the fall, autumn vegetables, including squash, pumpkin, and late-harvested potatoes, filled the back, with chrysanthemums in every color and size brightening the front.

One exceptionally warm morning in late spring, Martin, now seventy-two, was deciding on his project for the day. "The irises need to be divided," he told his wife. "You know, the ones against the south side of the house. The crop was really poor this year, and I suddenly realized that they've not been separated and thinned for almost seven years."

"That's nice, dear," his wife, Alice, muttered, as she worked on a fisherman-knit sweater for her newest son-in-law. "I never used to be able to knit in the hot weather," she said, "because of the way my hands used to sweat. Thank heavens for air-conditioning."

"That's nice, dear," Martin said, already planning where he would plant the leftover iris tubers. "You know, I think I'll see if Walter, next door, wants some of the extras."

"You do that," his wife said distractedly, using a tape measure to check the length of the sleeve she was knitting. She studied the pattern book. "Let's see. On this row I have to decrease five for the start of the underarm. And on the next row as well."

Martin heaved himself from his favorite lounge chair and started toward the door. "I'll see how many extra irises I have, then call Walter this evening. Those bearded dark purple ones would look real good beside the fence around his pool."

"That's good, dear. You do that," Alice said.

Martin walked out through the garage, where he put on his heavy gardening gloves. Because there were several bees' nests under the eaves of the house in the back, he wore an undershirt and a wool, long-sleeved shirt, briefs, and long work pants, with heavy wool socks and work boots. He walked around to the back of the house and crouched beside the thick row of iris foliage against the foundation. Slowly he pushed the topsoil from around the first few iris plants and worked his gloved fingers into the dirt.

It took two hours to pull up the first foot of plants. Now he had several dozen iris tubers, with neatly clipped wide, flat leaves attached. "Whew, it's getting hot," he muttered, looking at the sun, now high in the sky and beating on his back. Never known to sweat much, Martin wasn't particularly bothered by the heat.

Another hour passed and his wife called out and asked whether he wanted lunch. "I think I'll finish another section before I stop," he called back, then continued to work in the soil.

"Drink?"

"No, thanks," he said, returning to his irises.

As he worked, his breathing quickened, his heart rate increased, and his face became cool and clammy. His vision began to blur and he felt faint. Alarmed at how awful he suddenly felt, he tried to summon his wife. "Alice," he called softly. Knowing that she wouldn't be able to hear him from inside the house he stood up, staggered for a few steps, swayed, and fell to his knees. "Alice," he called again. He fell onto his side between two blueberry bushes.

"Fairfax Police to the ambulance. The rig is needed at 1424 Oak Hill for a possible heart attack. The caller's hysterical and says her husband is not breathing."

"10–4. 45–01 is responding."

Since I had had some quiet work to do, I had decided to pick up some extra hours riding the noon-to-six shift. I had closeted myself in the office at the back of the FVAC garage and had been trying to balance my checkbook for an hour. I was still off by one hundred dollars.

Since we had been told that we had a possible cardiac arrest, I was grateful that we had a full duty crew that day. Pete Williamson, a professional paramedic, was our crew chief, Dave Hancock was our driver, and Tim Babbett, just eighteen and not yet an EMT, was riding as a fourth. If we had to run a code we'd need all the trained hands we could get.

We sped toward the scene with Dave and Pete in front and Tim and me in the back. "Tim," I said, mentally assembling the equipment we might need, "as soon as we stop, I'll get the megaduffel and you put the defibrillator and the suction unit on the stretcher. Then we'll strap it all down." In addition to BP cuff, stethoscope, and trauma supplies, the megaduffel contained oxygen equipment, airways, and a bag-valve-mask in case we needed to artificially ventilate our patient.

As Tim started to move, I cautioned, "Wait for the rig to stop. It's not safe climbing around while we go lights and siren. Sit down and buckle up. Then we'll both move when the rig stops."

I felt the rig slow and turn into a driveway. As we came to a stop, Tim and I quickly loaded the stretcher so that when Dave opened the back doors, we could take out all the equipment at once. Dave would get a long backboard from the side compartment and follow us.

"Back here," I heard a woman yell. "In the back, in the garden. I think he stopped breathing."

Tim and I ran around the house pulling the stretcher, following Pete who was in turn following a gray-haired woman. As we rounded the corner of the house, I watched Pete kneel beside the supine man. "What's the story?" he asked Chuck Harding, the Fairfax police officer who was checking the man's carotid pulse.

"I just got here myself. He's totally unresponsive and I don't think he's breathing," the cop said. "His wife says she found him like this when she tried to call him for lunch."

Pete banged on the man's shoulder. "Can you hear me?" He got no response.

"He's so still," his wife said, wringing her hands. "I couldn't see his chest moving. Is he having a heart attack?"

"Just calm down," I told her, my arm on her shoulder, "and let us examine him." Reluctantly she stepped back out of our way and burst into tears.

Chuck backed up while Pete bent down and, with his ear near the man's mouth and his fingers on his neck, checked the man's vital signs. "He's got a pulse but he's not breathing."

I had already connected the BVM to the oxygen tank and I had the flow meter on full. Tim handed a medium airway to Pete, who quickly sized it against the man's face.

"What's his name, ma'am?" Pete asked.

"Martin," the woman said loudly through her tears. "His name's Martin."

"Martin," Pete said into the man's ear. "We're here to help you." I watched Pete insert the airway into the man's mouth to hold his tongue out of the way. Had he been at all responsive, he wouldn't have tolerated the airway and would have gagged.

"Any heart history?" I asked the woman.

"No, none. He's always been so healthy. He was working on his irises. The bearded purple ones." Her voice faded.

Pete fitted the mask of the BVM over Martin's mouth and nose, lifted his chin, and squeezed the bag. We could see the man's chest rise and fall. "Tim, take over bagging. Joan, get his shirt open so we can get an EKG," Pete yelled. I bent down and unbuttoned the man's shirt.

"I wonder why he's wearing this heavy flannel," I muttered. I opened his shirt and raised his undershirt to expose his chest. His chest was red and hot to the touch. "Pete, he's burning up."

Tim took over the mask-seal and Chuck squeezed the bag, forcing life-saving oxygen into Martin's lungs, Pete shifted around and touched the patient's chest. "Holy shit, he's so hot." He turned to Dave, who was standing with the longboard ready for use. "Get me several cold packs, three or four towels, and a bottle of sterile water. This may not be heart at all. I think he's suffering from the heat."

As Dave sprinted to the rig, Pete said, "Joan, get his

shoes and socks off, then we'll remove his pants. I'll set up the defibrillator."

Tim and Chuck gave Martin a few more breaths, then Tim checked his respirations again. "He's breathing, but just barely. I'd say rate about eight per minute and shallow."

"Continue bagging at about twenty breaths per minute and monitor his rate. If it's heat, he should start to come around when we get him cooled down. Damn," Pete muttered, "I wish I could start a line." Although Pete's a paramedic, when he's not riding with an advanced life-support unit like Prescott's fly car, he can function only as an EMT.

"Will he be okay?" his wife asked.

"We're doing everything we can to help him," I said, not really knowing the answer to her question.

Unable to deal with the heavy work boots, I finally abandoned the task of removing the man's shoes and used my heavy EMT shears to cut up the front of his pants legs.

"I'm going to use the small electrodes," Pete said. "He's got a weak pulse right now. Let's hope we won't need anything more." The small pads are used for monitoring, the large ones for delivering a shock to a heart that has stopped beating.

As Pete completed the connections, Dave returned with cold packs, water, and towels.

"I see sinus tach at about 210," Pete said. Sinus tachycardia indicated that Martin's heart was beating very quickly. Whereas a normal heart beats at between 60 and 80 beats per minute, Martin's heart was racing at about three times that fast. "The rhythm's regular, no PVCs." PVCs, or premature ventricular contractions, are occasional irregular beats that indicate that a heart is in deep trouble. Martin's heart was overworked but holding its own.

"Dave," Pete said, "put cold packs in the man's groin, under his arms, and across his throat." Dave punched the first cold pack to release the blue liquid chemical that would combine with the crystals and make the plastic bag cold.

"Joan, you can disconnect the defibrillator so we can cool him down." I unsnapped the wire leads, took the towels that Dave had brought, and laid one across the man's chest, working around the electrodes. "Pull off the electrodes if you have to," Pete said to me.

I unscrewed the top from the bottle of sterile water and poured half the contents onto the towel. I opened Martin's pants, draped a second towel across his abdomen, and poured water on it as well.

Tim disconnected the BVM from the oxygen and replaced it with a non-rebreather face mask. "He's breathing on his own now," he said as he fastened the oxygen mask over Martin's face. "About twenty-four." By removing his heavy clothes and exposing him to the air, his overheated body was already cooling. The water would cool him even faster.

"Oh, my God," his wife said, "what's happening?"

I looked up at the distraught woman and said, "Your husband got too hot. We're cooling him down."

While Dave put a cold pack under each of the man's arms, Pete yelled, "Tim, get the board ready. We'll use it to lift him onto the stretcher."

Tim positioned the board against Martin's side, then opened the collar bag and readied the straps we would use to secure him to the board. We transferred Martin to the longboard and onto the stretcher. En route to the hospital, we continued to wet him down and watched his condition steadily improve.

At the hospital, Martin's temperature was measured at 104 degrees. "Imagine what it was when we arrived in his yard," I said, shaking my head.

Pete looked up from his paperwork. "Another few minutes and he would have been beyond help. His brain would have cooked."

Before we left the hospital, I stuck my head into Martin's cubicle. He was now fully alert, sitting up with a nasal canula delivering oxygen to his body. "What happened?" he asked me.

"You got overheated and you weren't drinking enough water. Too much sun and too many heavy clothes. Feeling better?"

"Yeah. I really am. It was pretty close, huh?"

"Pretty close. But you're well on the way to recovery."

Sometimes two heads are better than one. It's wonderful how, with combined experience and guesswork, two EMTs occasionally can diagnose something that neither can believe.

The ambulance had been dispatched for a possible drug overdose. As Linda Potemski, Nick Abrams, and I entered the living room of the large, well-maintained house, I could see patrol officer Will McAndrews talking to a teenage boy who was sitting on the sofa, staring blankly into space. A middle-aged couple, looking distraught, stood nearby watching.

"Look, Steve," Will was saying. "I'm not going to bust you. But we need to know what you're on."

"Nuthin'," the boy muttered sleepily.

Will saw us coming in and walked over to us before we got to the boy. "The boy's name is Steve Simmons. His father was sitting here watching TV and the boy was in his room down the hall, studying. His father told me that the boy came stumbling into the living room, bumping into things and mumbling to himself. The boy denies taking any drugs and his parents swear that he doesn't do drugs. He sure looks like he's into something, but I'm getting nowhere."

"Okay. Let us check him out alone," I said.

Knowing that sometimes medical people can get information that a cop can't, Will took the boy's parents out of the room, hoping I could find out what Steve had taken.

"Hi, I'm Joan," I said to the boy as we approached. "And this is Linda and Nick." I nodded toward my crew. "How're you doing?"

"All right," he mumbled.

"Do you know where you are?" I asked.

The boy stared at me silently.

"Listen, Steve, we're not cops, and we need to know what you have taken in order to help you."

"Taken nothin'," Steve mumbled as his head nodded forward, then jerked upward.

"Steve, we're going to examine you. Okay?"

" 'Kay," he replied.

We quickly checked his vital signs but found nothing out of the ordinary. His pulse was a little slow and his pupil response to light was a little sluggish, but there was nothing that would indicate a drug overdose. He had good sensation and equal, if weak, strength in both hands and feet, no indication of any type of brain disease or injury. But he was confused, disoriented, and nodding out. Something was obviously seriously wrong.

"Why don't you get the stretcher," I said to Linda and Nick, then turned back to Steve. "We're going to take you over to the hospital to find out what's wrong with you. Okay?"

" 'Kay."

Steve was cooperative but his mind was pretty well scrambled as we got him on the stretcher and wheeled him out to the ambulance. I asked Linda to drive code 3, with lights and siren. As we began to roll toward the hospital, Nick said, "Maybe we ought to put him on oxygen."

"Sure, why not?" I replied, only because I couldn't think of anything else to do for the boy. The oxygen wouldn't hurt him and maybe, somehow, it would help.

Nick turned on the onboard oxygen tank, hooked it to

an oxygen mask, set the liter flow to 10, and put the mask over the boy's face. Then he moved around so he could monitor Steve's condition.

"Maybe he has a fever," I suggested, grasping at straws to explain the boy's illness. But Nick, who was holding Steve's hand and talking to him, trying to reassure him, said, "No, I don't think so. His hand is cold. As a matter of fact, it's like ice."

Although we carry disposable plastic fever thermometers on the rig, we rarely use them. Checking for fever is not a routine part of our examination protocol, except occasionally for a child having convulsions, a situation commonly caused by a high temperature. But since I didn't know what else to do, I reached into the supply cabinet, took out a plastic thermometer, snapped off the top, and put the underlying strip with its printed dots in the boy's mouth.

After a couple of minutes, I removed the thermometer and looked at the color of the dots. The more red dots on the strip, the higher the fever. But all of the dots were black. The thermometer didn't even show three red dots, the indicator of normal temperature.

"There must be something wrong with this thermometer," I said. "It's not working." I got up, took out another one, and repeated the procedure to check Steve's temperature. Again, all of the dots were black. I handed the thermometer to Nick. "Look at this. I've never seen anything like it."

Nick stared at the strip. "It's not recording any temperature. It's as if his body temperature were too low to record. Could he be hypothermic? Without being cold? In his own house?"

"I've never heard of it," I said, shaking my head, "but let's treat it like it might be true." We didn't know how or why, but Steve's body temperature had fallen to a dangerous level.

"Get the heater on," I said. "Full blast. I'll get some blankets and hot packs." As Nick cranked the heat up,

I reached over Steve, opened the bin next to the stretcher, and pulled out three plastic bags. I activated the heat packs, put one against Steve's chest and one under each arm, then covered him with every blanket in the rig.

"Linda ought to turn off her lights and siren and take it code 2," I said to Nick. "If he's seriously hypothermic, the bouncing of the ambulance can cause his heart to go into ventricular fibrillation. As a matter of fact, we should tell Linda to go slowly yet as efficiently as possible."

With agonizing frustration we crawled toward the hospital, sweating in the overheated ambulance. By the time we reached Fairfax General, Steve was showing a marked improvement.

"What happened?" he asked as we wheeled him into the emergency room.

"We're not sure," I said, "but we think your body temperature dropped very low."

"Cold?" he asked. "It's not winter. I don't understand."

"Neither do we," I said, "but you certainly seem to be feeling a lot better. I'm sure that the doctor will tell you what happened." I winked. "Then he can tell us."

I checked with the hospital a week later. Steve had been admitted, then discharged a few days later. As he and his parents had told us, he had taken no drugs. Rather, he was diagnosed as having had an unusual type of seizure disorder. Unlike most seizures, caused by electrical activity in the brain that results in unconsciousness and convulsions, Steve's episode had disrupted his brain's ability to regulate his body temperature and he had nearly died of hypothermia in his normally heated home during the summer. I understand his condition will respond to medication.

When we respond to a call, we never know what kind of a situation we will be thrown into.

* * *

It was the middle of the night, and Ed and I had been
called to meet the ambulance at the home of a forty-
five-year-old woman who, according to the police dispatcher, was having a heart attack. Since Bob Fiorella
was on vacation, Sam Middleton was our driver. He
was also riding from his home and, since he lived
around the corner from headquarters, he would pick up
the ambulance.

We found the woman sitting on a couch, clutching
her arm. She told us her name was Maria McMillan.

"I was making a midnight snack," she told me,
"when I got this pain in my left arm and shoulder. I'm
having a heart attack, I know it."

"Did you break into a sweat when the pain started?"
I asked, checking for the other signs and symptoms of
a heart attack.

"No," she answered.

"Any dizziness or nausea?"

"No. But my father died of a heart attack when he
was just fifty-five."

Ed had hooked up the police officer's oxygen tank
and placed a mask over her nose and mouth. The rest
of her words were muffled as she breathed pure oxygen.

"Are you having any other pain or any trouble
breathing?"

"Not really, but the pain's radiating from my shoulder
to my arm. My fingers are getting numb."

"All right," I said, skeptical about the cause of her
pain. "We'll take you over to the hospital and let the
doctors take a look at you."

My radio came to life. "45–01 to FPD. I'm on location." I recognized Sam's voice and keyed my radio.
"We just need the stretcher," I said.

While Ed went outside to help get the stretcher, I
used the equipment in Ed's crash kit to take a set of vitals. "Are you taking any medications?" I asked.

"I take something for my high blood pressure," she said, "and I take lithium."

Lithium, I knew, was frequently prescribed to treat depression. I stored that fact for entry into my report. I finished taking her BP. "Your blood pressure is 170 over 100," I said. "That's a bit high. Did you take your medications today?"

"Yes," she said.

As I made notes on a piece of paper for later transcription to the prehospital care report, I looked at the arm she was holding. It was her right. "You know," I said, "I'm right-left stupid. When someone tells me to raise my right hand, I make a random decision." I paused. "Aren't you holding your right arm? Is it your left or right that's giving you the trouble?" Cardiac pain is traditionally thought to radiate down the left arm, but in unusual cases it does travel down the right. I needed to know for my report.

Mrs. McMillan looked down, puzzled. Then, with as little movement as possible, she switched her hands so she was holding her left arm. "Left. That's the heart attack side and this is a heart attack. I know it."

"Of course," I answered. Something was very wrong here, but thank heavens it wasn't my job to find out what.

"Is that oxygen mask comfortable?" I knew that the oxygen would do no harm and might allay some of her fears.

"It's all right. And where's Betty?"

"Betty?"

"My daughter." The woman became agitated. "Betty!"

"I'm right here, Mom," a voice said. A nice-looking young woman in her early twenties rose from a chair in the corner of the room. She looked frazzled and bewildered. "I'm just staying out of the way."

The woman relaxed markedly. "You'll come with me," she said.

"Of course, Mom. I'm very worried about you."

Ed and Sam returned with the stretcher and we settled the woman comfortably onto it. We lifted the stretcher into the rig and while Ed and I rode in the back, Mrs. McMillan's daughter rode in the front, with Sam.

"Mrs. McMillan," I said when we were on the way to the hospital, "how's the pain now?"

"Much better." She leaned over, close to me. "You know, maybe I'm not having a heart attack."

Not knowing what to answer, I remained silent.

"It's important that I get Betty to the hospital, but I didn't want to tell her about it. It might frighten her."

"Tell her about what?" I inquired.

"The drugs, of course."

"Which drugs?" I asked. I had no idea what was going on, but the woman wanted to talk and I wanted to keep her as calm as I could until we reached the hospital.

"The ones they're feeding her so she will go along quietly."

"Go along? To where?"

"Why, to Arabia. They're white slavers and they're going to take Betty to Arabia where she'll become the concubine of some sultan." She leaned closer to my ear. "They love blondes, you know." I remembered that Betty's hair was ash blond.

"Really?"

"Of course. Everyone knows that. That's why they picked her. So now they're sneaking drugs into her food. It's a miracle that I haven't swallowed any, but I'm very careful about what I eat."

"I see," I said, not knowing what else to say.

"So, you can understand, I'm sure, that I had to do something to get her to the hospital so she can be tested for drugs. Then she'll believe me."

"She doesn't believe you about this?"

"No. Do you have any children?"

"Two girls," I answered. "Grown and living far away."

"Well, with two girls I'm sure you understand what a mother goes through."

"It's not easy being a mother," I said, making what conversation I could. The hospital would have to sort this all out.

As Mrs. McMillan continued, I felt the rig turn into the hospital parking bay. We removed the oxygen and wheeled our patient into the emergency room. When she was settled in a cubicle, I quickly recapped the story she had told me to Dr. Margolis, the doctor in charge. "It sounds like she needs psychiatric help," he said. "Joan, would you mind talking to the daughter? Find out who her doctor is, her psychiatric history, and whatever else seems relevant. We're very short-staffed and you seem to have a handle on what's happening. Maybe you can get us started."

I found Betty in the waiting room. "Betty," I said, "your mother's very worried about you."

"Is she having a heart attack?"

"I don't think so. She seems to be more concerned about you."

"Did she tell you the drug thing?" she asked softly. "Yes."

"She hasn't eaten much for weeks. She's convinced that someone's trying to drug me." Betty opened her purse and pulled out a crumpled tissue. "I have no idea where she got that idea from, but now she only eats what she can prepare from unopened cans and boxes. Once a box of cereal is opened, we eat from it while she watches the package, then she throws it out. And she won't let me out of her sight."

"I think she needs help," I said.

"I know. She was seeing a shrink, but she stopped seeing him about six months ago. Things have gotten much worse."

"Do you remember the name of the doctor she was seeing?"

"I can look it up." She rummaged in her purse and pulled out two prescription bottles. "I brought her medications. Her blood pressure medication is from her regular doctor," she said, dropping one bottle back into her purse, "but the lithium is from Dr. . . ." She examined the label. ". . . Bennett, in Davenport, I think."

"Okay, I'll give this information to the doctor and he'll decide whether to contact Dr. Bennett. Just relax. The hospital will see that your mother gets the help she needs. Are you okay?"

"I'm holding together. Will they take good care of my mother?"

"Of course. I'll tell Dr. Margolis you're here and he'll come out and talk to you shortly."

I relayed what Betty had told me to Dr. Margolis. "Thanks, Joan," he said. "We'll take it from here. I'll contact Harry Bennett and have him come over."

As we left the hospital, I told the story to Ed and Sam. "God damn. Don't you get pissed as shit at people who use us this way?" Sam asked. "She didn't have any reason to call an ambulance. Call a cab. Call a shrink. That's my advice. We're not a taxi service for wackos."

I thought about not saying what was on my mind since I know that many people in the corps feel the way Sam does. But I had to disagree. "You know," I said, "I guess I don't care if the illness is in the body or the mind. She was just as sick in her own way as someone having a diabetic reaction. I just hope she'll get the help she needs."

Sam made a rude noise. "She should have taken a taxi and not jerked our chains."

I just hope that I made her trip to the hospital a little easier.

Short Subjects

People respond in the most amazing ways when they're caught in an emergency situation.

Ed and I had a call for a woman having severe abdominal pain. When we arrived at her home, we were assaulted by the smell of our obviously incontinent patient. She was semiconscious, reeking of urine and feces. Her daughter, hovering in the background, gave us what information we needed.

We checked the older woman out, took a quick set of vitals, and transferred her to our stretcher while the daughter stood silently outside the doorway of the sickroom.

As we wheeled our patient out the front door, her daughter ran alongside the stretcher with a perfume atomizer, squirting the sheets and the air around us.

The call was for a woman with an allergic reaction at Hair Event, a local beauty parlor. When we arrived the woman was sitting in one of the operator's chairs, her hair soaking wet and drooping into her face. She was having respiratory problems. "It must be the pine nuts," she told us. "I've had trouble like this before."

"I never suspected you were allergic," the hairstylist said. "Those cookies come from the local Italian bakery and certainly could have had pine nuts in them."

"I can't go yet," the woman said as I took her blood pressure. "My hair." I could hear odd squeaking noises when she breathed.

"Ma'am," I said. "You need a shot of adrenaline for your allergy. And you need it quickly." A severe reaction like this could cause respiratory arrest and death.

"But my hair." She tried to catch her breath. "I'll look a fright."

It took several precious moments of argument before

her hairstylist agreed to fit her in at any time to finish her shampoo, cut, and blow dry. With that assurance she agreed to be transported.

On another occasion, we picked up a woman who was also having breathing problems, this time due to a severe asthma attack. Her breathing was noisy and I didn't have to use my stethoscope to hear her wheezing.

"Where's your inhaler?" I asked her, knowing she must have one with her history of asthma.

"It's empty," she puffed. "I meant to have the prescription refilled—" Puff, puff. "—but I never got around to it." We put her on high-flow oxygen, sat her fully upright, and loaded her into the ambulance. "I want to go to St. Luke's," she whispered, her condition worsening with every minute that passed.

"I want you to go to the closest hospital and Fairfax General is only four minutes away." As I spoke we transferred her to the life-giving oxygen of our onboard tank.

"But my doctor's at St. Luke's," she wheezed.

"We can't wait. You need medications I don't have." I stuck my head through the opening and told the driver to drive, code 3, to Fairfax General.

As we pulled out of the driveway and headed down Route 10, our patient was sitting bolt upright, breathing as much oxygen as she could and looking idly out the back window. As we drove down Route 10, we saw a car speed across an intersection behind us, going the other way.

The woman pushed her mask aside. "Oh, no." She moaned, shaking her head. "That was my husband. I forgot that I told him to meet me at St. Luke's." Weakly she waved out the back window at the disappearing vehicle. "He's going to the wrong hospital."

We arrived at the driver's side of a car that had been involved in a one-car accident. We could see that the driver was unconscious with serious head and chest injuries where his unseatbelted body had smashed into the steering wheel and windshield. As I pressed my hand against his head to keep him from moving, he regained consciousness and began to yell.

"Where's Molly?" he screamed. We tried to restrain him with only limited success. "Find Molly! Help her!" He lapsed into unconsciousness.

"Who's Molly?" I yelled. When I got no response, I took a quick glance around inside the car. I didn't see any car seat, dolls, or blankets. Molly, and all her things, must have been thrown from the vehicle, I thought. "We've got a missing child," I yelled. "Look around carefully. I've got no age or description."

As the crew and bystanders fanned out to search, I tried to get information from the driver. "Sir, how old's the child?"

He moaned. "Not child. It's my dog. She's a cocker spaniel. She was in the back." He tried to wriggle around to see into the backseat.

"Sir, you have to hold still," I said. I looked onto the back floor and I saw the bloody body of a dog, wedged under the front seat. He saw it too. "Take care of Molly," he screamed. "I won't let you take care of me unless you fix Molly."

"Sir," I argued. "Let us care for you first, then we'll take care of Molly."

"Her first. I can refuse treatment, and I will unless you fix Molly."

We called off the search for the missing child. One of our EMTs and two firefighters took charge of the dog, carefully placing her on a short backboard and sliding her out of the car. As we immobilized the driver, he watched the team bandage the dog, arrange oxygen tubing so she would get as much oxygen as she could and slide the animal, board and all, into a chief's car.

"Take her in the ambulance," the man cried.

"Can't do that," I said. "The health department, our insurance company, and our rules won't allow it. Molly's comfortable now, and they'll take her to the animal hospital. They've got someone on call twenty-four hours a day. Meanwhile, let's get you taken care of."

"Are you sure she'll be okay?"

"I have no idea," I answered truthfully, "but I know she'll get good care."

I got a note a few weeks later. Both the driver and the dog survived the accident, battered but now recovering at home. Whenever I think about this call I remember a comment my mother used to make. She used to say, "When you hear hoofbeats, assume horses." But sometimes they're really zebras.

One afternoon, we were on our way to the hospital with our patient, a man of at least seventy. He was suffering from some difficulty breathing, but he was conscious and alert. I had reviewed his medical history with him, and he had told me about his cardiac problems and his two small strokes.

"Anything else I should know?" I asked.

"I suffer from all the things that old folks get," he said to me. "And I have CRS."

I racked my brain, not wanting to appear ignorant, but I came up with no condition called CRS. So I asked. "What's CRS?"

"Oh," he said with a smile, "that's 'Can't Remember Shit.' "

Even the doctors at the hospital occasionally react in an unexpected way.

We brought a victim of an auto accident into the emergency room and, since the staff was very busy, I helped remove the last of the victim's clothes. As I cut the center of her 34DD bra, I was amazed at the way her breasts remained standing straight up. Some doctor had enhanced her shape with a great deal of silicone.

At that moment, in walked the straight-laced doctor who was, at that time, head of the ER staff. He looked at the face of our unconscious patient, then his gaze traveled lower. Softly he muttered, "Wow! Monstrous magumbas."

I managed to smother my laughter until I was out of the ER.

Chapter 6

Brian DeVry was proud of his vegetable garden. He had been expanding it year by year, and now it took up most of his backyard. Although he was largely an organic gardener, his quarter-acre yielded tomatoes, peas, three varieties of squash, string beans, broccoli, cauliflowers, and eggplants, as many as his family, friends, and neighbors could consume. He subscribed to several organic gardening magazines, and to improve his crop he had tried methods ranging from planting marigolds to buying praying mantis egg cases.

It was a hot day in mid-June and Brian was on his way back from the Lazy S stable. A couple of times a year, he drove his pickup truck to the stable and took as much raw horse manure as he wanted—for free. Back home, he would shovel it onto his compost heap and apply a high-nitrogen fertilizer between the layers. The heat of decomposition would make it steam for most of the winter, and by the following spring it would become a rich and valuable addition to his garden's soil.

As he drove along Route 10, his pickup truck was loaded with as much of the aromatic manure as he had been able to shovel in. It formed a small mountain in the back of the truck.

"I may have gotten carried away," Brian muttered to himself. "The truck handles like shit." He cackled at his choice of words.

Brian made a right onto Hunter's Hill Road and headed down the long grade toward Deerfield. Ahead, he saw the full stop at the Deerfield intersection and, as he had thousands of times before, he pressed his foot on the brake. The truck slowed but did not stop. Brian lifted his foot and pressed again. The truck slowed only a bit more. Brian glanced at the speedometer. Thirty-five. He pumped the brake but there was no response. As his brain whirled, trying to decide whether to try down-shifting, he caught a glimpse of a small red sports car approaching from his right.

He knew that there was no full stop on Deerfield, and since this section of Hunter's Hill was lightly traveled, most people tended to race through the intersection. He suspected that the driver mightn't think to look both ways, so he leaned on the horn. He saw no reaction from the woman who was driving. He could hear the loud radio music coming from the open car. She'll never hear me, he thought. "Lady, stop!" he screamed, banging his hand on the horn. "Stop!" As if in slow motion, Brian finally saw the woman glance to her left, but by then it was too late. Brian felt the impact of the collision and watched a waterfall of horse manure cascade over the roof of his truck and down his windshield.

Seventeen-year-old Marcy Hamilton loved her brother's two-seater Mazda and swapped her old clunker with him whenever she could. She loved to open the windows, turn the radio up loud, and drive around town "feeling the road." That morning, she had driven to her brother's house and left her eleven-year-old dark blue Chrysler in his driveway. She had "borrowed" her brother's car using her duplicate key, sped across town, and spent the morning with her boyfriend, Paul.

It was now almost noon and the temperature was already over ninety degrees. The sun was blazing, so Marcy opened all the windows and the sun roof as she drove toward the mall to pick up her dress for the junior prom. Then, reluctantly, she was going to return the car.

As she approached the Hunter's Hill intersection, "Rock Around the Clock" blared from her favorite oldies station. "Put your glad rags on," she sang, banging her hand on the steering wheel in rhythm with the song, "and join the fun." She heard a car horn and looked to her left, just in time to see the black pickup truck about five feet from her door. "Dear God," she screamed as the vehicles collided.

The call came into ambulance headquarters only moments after the accident. "Fairfax Police to the ambulance corps. An ambulance is needed at the intersection of Deerfield and Hunter's Hill for a PIAA."

A personal injury auto accident. It could be anything from no injuries to an MCI—a multiple casualty incident. Quickly Jack McCaffrey, Joan, and I jumped into the ambulance and sped, lights flashing and siren blaring, onto the northbound parkway.

We pulled off at the Hunter's Hill exit, drove until we saw the accident, and pulled the rig to a stop. A black pickup truck and a tiny red Mazda were locked together. Jack ran to check out the driver of the pickup, who was standing, talking to a policeman, while Joan and I walked around the front of the rig. "I'll check with the cops and survey the scene for any more victims," Joan said, wrinkling her nose.

"Good. I'll see who's in the Mazda."

"What's that stench?" Joan asked.

"Smells like manure," I said as I walked toward the tiny red car, puzzled.

I saw that the front end of the truck was embedded in the driver's-side door of the Mazda. The side of the sports car had been pushed into its passenger compartment—against the left side of the driver. I looked in through the windshield and saw a teenage girl, in tears, half buried in what looked and smelled like horse manure. In the fifteen years I had been volunteering with the Fairfax Volunteer Ambulance Corps, I had never been in a situation quite like this.

I went around to the passenger side and opened the Mazda's door. I almost gagged at the odor but I knew I had to get in. It's my job, not in a paid sense since we're all volunteers, but it was my responsibility. I had to help. I had no choice.

As I put my knee on the passenger seat, squooshing into a pile of manure, I thought, Why me? Pushing horseshit aside, I reached toward the sobbing girl.

"My name is Ed," I said, introducing myself as I always do when approaching a patient. "I'm with the Fairfax Ambulance Corps. What's your name?"

"Marcy," she cried. "I can't move. Get me out of here."

"We will, Marcy," I responded, "but first I have to know what happened and where you are hurt."

"I was on my way to pick up my prom dress and return this car to my brother. That truck came out of nowhere and hit me. I just got my driver's license a few months ago. My brother'll kill me."

"Where are you hurt, Marcy?"

"My left arm hurts and my left leg seems to be stuck. It only hurts a little but I can't move."

"Try not to move at all," I said, "especially your head and neck."

Marcy's face and chest appeared to be uninjured, and she seemed to be breathing easily. As far as I could see, there was no bleeding. Her skin color appeared normal.

"Are you having any trouble breathing?" I asked.

"No."

Through the lumps of manure, I examined her head, neck, back, and chest and found no obvious injury. I felt as much as I could of the left side of her body and again found nothing life-threatening.

I held two fingers of each hand out in front of her. "Please squeeze my fingers with both hands, Marcy," I requested. The pressure of both hands was equal.

Marcy was buried almost up to her knees. Hoping my latex gloves would protect me from the worst of the mess, I reached down and dug to her feet. I checked each foot and again found no sign of serious injury.

"The driver of the truck isn't hurt at all," I heard Joan say through Marcy's window, "and there are no more victims. The police have a tow truck coming, and the fire department's on the way in case we need extrication."

"Good. Marcy seems to be in pretty good shape," I said. "She's complaining of pain in her left arm and leg, but nothing too serious from what I can feel. But her left leg seems to be pinned so we'll need the Hurst Tool to get her out. I'll stay with Marcy while the fire department opens things up for us."

"Collar?" Joan asked.

"Medium," I said, gauging the size of Marcy's neck.

Joan handed me the appropriate-sized flexible plastic collar, and, with her help, I fastened it around Marcy's neck. "This is to remind you not to move your head and neck."

"Am I badly hurt?" Marcy asked.

"You're probably not hurt at all," I answered. "But we have to protect you, just in case. Our protocols say that we have to collar anyone who's been in an accident like this, just as a precaution."

"Okay. Whatever you say."

I saw the driver of the pickup truck approach the Mazda. "Are you okay?" he asked my patient. "Hey, I'm sorry, lady. My brakes gave out. I couldn't stop. I tried to warn you. I honked and honked. I guess you couldn't hear me." He turned to Jack who ran up behind him. "Is she going to be okay? I tried to warn her."

"Come on with me and sit in the ambulance," Jack said as he guided the uninjured driver away from the red car.

"I guess I had the radio up a little loud," Marcy said.

"I didn't hear a thing." She paused. "Boy, it really stinks in here. I'm afraid I may be sick."

The sun was acting on the manure, filling the car with fumes. "Don't you dare," I said, "because if you do, then I will and we'll both be in more of a mess than we are now."

Marcy smiled. "I'll try not to. You try too."

"Joan," I called, "get me the Vick's VapoRub."

"VapoRub? What for?" Marcy asked.

"You'll see." A few moments later Joan returned from the rig with the small blue jar in her hand. I took it from her and explained. "I'm going to put a little on my upper lip. Then all I'll smell is the menthol, not the . . ." I looked at the manure. Bits were still falling into the car from the roof. "Want some too?"

"Sure," Marcy said. Carefully, without moving Marcy's head, I put a dollop of Vick's on her upper lip and some on mine. "Better?"

"Yeah," Marcy said, sounding surprised. "It really is."

"That's great. Now, I know how much you want to get out of this mess, but I'm afraid it might take a little while. We're going to get you out safely and carefully, but I'll stay with you all the time and hold your head so you don't move. Okay?"

"Okay," Marcy said, seeming calmer and reassured. Moving just her eyes, she looked around the inside of the tiny car. "Oh, Lord," she moaned. "My brother's going to kill me."

It took about ten minutes for the fire department to stabilize the car and for a tow truck to slowly pull Brian's pickup truck away from Marcy's car. Then the firefighters covered Marcy and me with a tarp to protect us from flying glass and debris while they carefully removed the windshield and the rear window.

Despite the VapoRub, under the tarp the smell was almost overwhelming. Between that, the heat, and the darkness, Marcy began to panic. "Please get me out," she cried.

I spoke slowly and calmly. "We are going to get you out as quickly as possible, but first the firefighters have to get the door off the car. It's going to be noisy and you may feel the car move, but don't be scared. You're safe and I'm right here with you."

"But it's so dark," Marcy whimpered.

"This is just to protect us while the firefighters do their job," I explained. "I've done this dozens of times and I've never been hurt. I trust those guys. Will you trust them too?"

"I guess. But it's so scary."

"I know." Although I told Marcy the truth, and I have done it dozens of times, I've never gotten used to it. Being inside a car while it is being cut and pried apart, listening to the shouts of the firefighters, the sounds of the extrication tools, and the tearing and snapping of steel all around you is terrifying. So you talk, both to calm your patient and to try to control your own fear.

"Tell me about your dress," I asked.

As she started to describe her prom dress, a loud pulsing, churning sound began. I felt myself begin to sweat, as much from fear as from the hot, stagnant air under the tarp. The smell of gasoline exhaust fumes began to mix with the stench of the manure. After a few moments Marcy said, "I'm scared. What are they doing? When are they going to get me out?"

"Marcy, I know it's dark and scary and noisy down here and it's going to get noisier. Would you like me to tell you exactly what the firefighters are doing out there?"

"I guess. What's that noise?"

"The sound you hear now," I began, "is the gasoline-powered hydraulic pump that powers the Hurst Tool. You might know it as the jaws of life. They're going to use the jaws to pry the door off the car so they can get you out."

"I've seen that on TV," Marcy said. "Like in those rescue shows." We could hear the sound of metal tools and a slight creaking.

"That's right. Now they're using a large metal crowbar called a Halligan Tool to pry open a space near the door hinge so that they can insert the tip of the jaws. The jaws are like a giant pair of pliers, and in this case they're probably using them in reverse, to pry apart. Okay so far?" I wanted to keep her talking.

"I guess."

Despite the creaks and snaps, I continued my explanation, keeping my voice calm and even. "As the tip opens, it will bend the metal back until the door is forced off the hinges."

The car jolted slightly as the tip of the Hurst Tool was inserted into the small opening. Then the sounds of the jaws began. There was no vibration, just the straining and tearing of metal.

Suddenly there was a loud bang. In the darkness, it sounded like a gunshot. Marcy screamed.

"It's okay, Marcy," I reassured her. "That was the first door hinge letting go. There'll be another pop when they break the second hinge, then they'll be able to remove the door. But we may have to wait a little longer after that. They'll probably want to peel back the roof so that we have plenty of room to get you out."

The second hinge popped a few moments later. Within seconds I felt the tarp lifted from our bodies. "Are we done now?" Marcy asked.

"Seems so. Are you okay?"

Marcy smiled. "I think I am. I got through that in one piece."

Joan examined the now accessible left side of Marcy's body. "I'm going to have to cut away some of your clothing in order to examine you, Marcy," Joan said. "I'll tell the firefighters to move back so we can have some privacy. Okay?"

"Wait a minute," Marcy replied, a gleam in her eye.

"Maybe we should let them stay. Are any of them cute?"

Joan and I both smiled. We always consider it a job well done when the patient relaxes sufficiently to kid around.

After Joan completed her examination, she turned to me. "Her left arm, leg, and hip are bruised but there is no deformity and only a little swelling., I don't think anything is broken. What do you think? Should we extricate her through the door or have the firefighters peel back the roof?"

I cringed at the thought of getting back under the tarp, but even with the door off we had very little room for extrication and Marcy appeared to be stable. She could tolerate a few more minutes in the car.

"Let's get the roof off and do the job right," I replied. "All right with you, Marcy?"

"Yeah. But could I have some more of that VapoRub first?"

We dabbed more goo on our upper lips, then the firefighters covered us with the tarp again and began the process of peeling back the car roof.

"This won't take long," I reassured Marcy. "They are going to use a giant shearslike Hurst Tool attachment to cut through the posts that hold up the front of the roof. Then they'll simply bend the roof back to give us plenty of room to get you out."

This time there was little noise other than the throb of the pump motor as the giant shears easily cut through the two posts on either side of the windshield and then through the two posts behind the car doors. Within minutes the roof had been folded back and, even under the tarp, daylight filled the vehicle.

Suddenly the noise stopped and it was over. The tarp was taken away and we could begin to remove our patient from what was left of the car. It was interesting to watch my crew and the firefighters try to help without

touching the filthy patient or the horseshit-filled car unless absolutely necessary.

Despite the mess, we were soon en route to Fairfax
General Hospital.

At the hospital, after finishing my paperwork, I
walked over to Dr. Margolis, who had just examined
Marcy. "How is she?" I asked.

"Well, I'm a bit concerned that she may have a head
injury. We'll know more after I send her upstairs for a
skull series."

I was horrified. I thought that I had done a thorough
patient survey. There had been no sign of head trauma.
Her neurologic functions had all been normal. Her pupils had been equal and reactive to light. She denied
any loss of consciousness, and she had been fully alert
through the entire extrication procedure and the trip to
the hospital. I must have missed something obvious.

I was afraid to ask, but I had to know so that I would
not make the same mistake again. "Why do you suspect
head trauma?"

"Well, she appears to be very confused. Her recollec-
tion of the events following the accident doesn't make
sense. She told me that she remained in the car after the
accident. She even described the extrication. But it's obvious that she was thrown out of the car. She's completely covered with dirt . . . and whatever." He fanned
his face with his hand. "And the smell. . . . What did
she land in?"

Dr. Margolis and everyone else in the emergency
room stared at me as I began to laugh. I had not made
a mistake in examining my patient, but I had forgotten
to communicate a key piece of information to the emergency room personnel. When I was able to stop laughing, I told Dr. Margolis about the horseshit that had
filled the car. "Maybe you don't have to bother with the
skull series after all," I suggested.

Marcy was lucky. She was treated and released the

same day. I was not so lucky. To this day, Dr. Margolis still teases me about my "horseshit call."

Most people who are involved in volunteer ambulance work truly want to provide sick or injured people with the best possible emergency medical care. But there is also a feeling of territoriality, of turf, and police or 911 dispatchers must be careful about dispatching the "correct" agency for fear of offending a volunteer group by sending "outside" rescuers into their district, even when the neighboring agency can respond faster. The problem is made worse by differences in the type of emergency medical response between districts in our state.

Emergency medical response in the Fairfax district is supplied by FVAC, an independent volunteer ambulance corps that provides patient care and the immobilization and removal of patients from vehicles. For all other rescue work, including cutting up cars and removal of patients from dangerous situations, FVAC depends on the Fairfax Fire Department.

FVAC is run in an almost military manner. Rules and standards are strictly enforced, with suspension or expulsion being the ultimate threat for serious infractions of the service rules or bylaws. Much of the time FVAC has full crews on duty at their headquarters. This allows a very short response time.

The Prescott Rescue Squad, a branch of the Prescott Volunteer Fire Association, provides the emergency medical response for the adjacent Prescott fire district. All of the Prescott Rescue Squad members have at least some training in rescue and firefighting as well as in patient care.

Although the general level of patient care in Prescott is excellent, there is greater variability than in FVAC, since some of the Prescott Rescue Squad members consider firefighting to be their primary interest. Discipline is more difficult to maintain because Rescue Squad members can still serve as firefighters even after suspension or expulsion from the Rescue Squad.

The Prescott Rescue Squad, however, tends to be a more closely knit group and its integrated fire-rescue-ambulance functions tend to make it more effective than FVAC at the scene of a major motor vehicle accident, fire, or other disaster. Although Prescott does not have full crews available at the firehouse as many hours as does FVAC, its crews assemble quickly when alerted by its pager system. Also, paid professional firefighter-EMTs, on duty at the firehouse, respond to the scene of medical emergencies with a fire engine. Thus, trained EMT response is very rapid although there is sometimes a delay in transport while volunteer crews assemble.

Prescott recently instituted a program in which a paid paramedic responds in a fly car to the scene of every ambulance call to provide advanced life support for the patient, if needed. Although an EMT can splint a broken bone, stop bleeding, extricate a patient from a crushed automobile, deliver a baby, and defibrillate a stopped heart, a paramedic also can start an IV line, administer drugs, and insert a tube down a patient's throat to assist breathing.

Over the years, the mode-of-operation differences and the social-historical differences (for over a hundred years, volunteer fire departments in our state have been exclusively men's social as well as service organizations whereas FVAC was founded only thirty years ago and is staffed by as many women as men) have resulted in misunderstandings and rivalry between the two neighboring services.

I recently joined Prescott Rescue, since I live in their district. I also remain an active member of FVAC. As a member of both organizations, I have to be very careful about using the correct color of emergency light when responding to a call: blue light for Prescott since it's technically a fire department and green for Fairfax Ambulance. Using the wrong light would be considered an almost unforgivable insult.

But there is also a great deal of cooperation between Prescott and FVAC, including joint quality-control call-review sessions, disaster drills, training meetings, and occasional social functions.

On one stretch of the parkway that forms the border between the two districts, between Route 10 and Hunter's Hill Road, the two agencies have agreed to a joint response because of the frequency and seriousness of the accidents that occur on the narrow, curved, and improperly banked road, and because usually it is easier for FVAC to get to the northbound lanes while the southbound lanes are more accessible to Prescott.

Although the parkway is under the jurisdiction of the state police, only a few patrol cars cover many miles of parkway; therefore, both Prescott and Fairfax police often respond until the state police arrive.

It was a mild evening in early April. Larry Wilcox had taken his three sons, Art, nine, Jim, twelve, and Larry Jr., seventeen, up to Whitehead Mountain for a day of skiing. It would probably be the last skiing of the season. It had been a glorious, crystal-clear day, and, although the spring snow had been less than wonderful, the lift lines had been shorter than they had been all winter. Most skiers probably have given up until next year, Larry thought.

They had skied all day and now they were on their way home, tired but content after a wonderful day. Larry was driving at the speed limit, carefully negotiating the curve on which, he knew from past experience, it was surprisingly difficult to keep the car from veering to the right. Suddenly Larry heard a bang and had to struggle to maintain control of his vehicle. Gently pumping his brakes, he slowed the car down, then pulled off the road onto what was now, due to the spring thaw, a sea of mud. He felt the wheels of his car sink into the ooze as he lurched to a stop.

Larry switched on his four-way flashers and stepped out, up to his ankles in muck. "I'm going to need a tow truck to get out of his," he yelled to the boys. Silently the three boys sulked in the backseat.

It was almost dark and cars were speeding past. Larry cursed himself for not having bought the flares that he knew he should have in his car for just such a situation. He walked up the road until he came to a mud-free shoulder, faced the oncoming traffic, and waved his hands over his head.

After what seemed like hours, a station wagon pulled over onto the relatively solid shoulder in front of him. Larry ran up to the wagon and found that the driver had opened the passenger-side window just a crack. He pointed toward his car, off the road. "My car's stuck in the mud," he yelled.

Through the slightly open window he heard a woman's voice. "What did you say?"

"My car's stuck in mud," he repeated. "I need help."

"What?" she repeated.

"Mud; mud; my car's in the mud," Larry yelled in frustration over the sound of the other vehicles speeding past.

Without a further word the woman sped off.

Leslie Hooper had hesitated to stop when she saw the man at the side of the road, frantically waving his hands. Just yesterday she had read about a car-jacking in a nearby small suburban town. Oh, what the hell, she thought. He looks like he's in trouble. She could see the taillights of what she assumed was Larry's car flashing up ahead. I'll keep my doors locked and just crack my window to find out what happened.

She pulled over onto the shoulder. As the man approached, she tapped the button that controlled the passenger-side window, lowering it just enough to hear him. But he seemed to become agitated and hostile as she tried to find out what the problem was. All she could make out was something about blood. She started to get spooked.

As Leslie pulled out onto the parkway, she picked up her cellular phone and dialed 911 to report a car off the road and something about blood.

At FVAC headquarters the klaxon sounded. "Fairfax Police to Fairfax Ambulance."

The Fairfax crew had just started dinner. Tom Franks groaned as he got up and walked to the radio. "They must know when we're eating," he complained.

"Ambulance on," he replied somewhat sullenly into the microphone.

"The ambulance is needed for a PIAA on the parkway southbound between Route 161 and Hunter's Hill Road. We have a report of someone bleeding seriously."

"That's a dual response area," Mike advised. "Dispatch Prescott Rescue also."

"10–4. Will do."

"Also, put the chopper on standby."

"10–4," the dispatcher answered.

"Fairfax Ambulance is responding to the southbound lane of the parkway between Route 161 and Hunter's Hill."

The Fairfax crew reluctantly left their dinner to get cold and sped toward the parkway, siren screaming and red and white lights flashing.

Hernandez Towing was new in town and was struggling to make its place in Fairfax. Known affectionately as You-Maul-We-Haul Towing, it had a garage on Hunter's Hill Road near the parkway. Tim Hernandez heard the ambulance dispatched on his scanner.

"Hey, Joe," he yelled to his mechanic, "get in the truck and get over to the parkway before General Towing beats us to the wreck." Joe got in the tow truck, switched on the yellow strobes, and headed toward the parkway.

State Police officer Sally Johnson was on the south-bound parkway about fifteen miles north of Larry's bogged-down car when she was dispatched to the "serious motor vehicle accident." She flipped on her lights and siren as she pressed down on the gas pedal.

Fairfax officer Will McAndrews received the dispatch as he was patrolling Deerfield Street near Hunter's Hill. His dispatcher told him that the State Police would be delayed because they had no patrol car nearby so he should check it out and see if he could be of assistance.

Will switched on his emergency lights and siren and headed toward the parkway. He would probably be first on the scene, which was only about two or three minutes away.

Prescott Patrol Officer Roy Zimmerman's radio awoke. "325 to 703."

"703."

"Respond to the southbound parkway between 161 and Hunter's Hill for a 10–2. Report of multiple severe injuries. State Police advises they will be delayed. I've got both Fairfax and Prescott ambulances responding."

"703. 10–4," Roy replied as his emergency lights and siren began to pierce the twilight.

I was just pulling out of the Three-Square Mini-Mart, where I had picked up a container of milk and some bagels for the following morning's breakfast, when my Prescott pager began to beep.

"GVK–861 Prescott to the Rescue Squad. Be advised, engine 722 and the rescue are responding with a full crew to a PIAA on the parkway, southbound, between Route 161 and Hunter's Hill."

Even though they had a full crew on the ambulance,

I was a lot closer to the scene and Prescott encouraged its members to respond, reasoning that extra help is always better than not enough help. I plugged in my blue emergency light and headed up Deerfield toward the parkway.

As I approached the scene, I could see Will McAndrews flaring out the right lane behind his patrol car. I saw that no ambulance or car with green or blue light had arrived yet. That meant that I would be the first EMT on the scene, a situation that I hated. No matter how much training and experience you've had, dealing with a serious medical emergency, possibly involving multiple victims, with no backup can be overwhelming.

I pulled over in front of the police car, which was parked on the pavement beside a car that was up to its floorboards in mud. I popped open my trunk, grabbed my trauma kit, and squooshed through the mud to the car, which appeared to be undamaged. I looked around for another vehicle but could see nothing.

A man and three boys stood on a low embankment away from the road. I walked over to the group, trying to keep out of as much of the mud as possible. "Are you hurt?" I asked.

"No," the man answered.

"Are there any other cars involved?" Will asked, approaching through the goo.

"No, just us. My car's stuck in the mud," the man replied.

"There's no accident? Nobody's hurt?" I asked again.

"No," Larry replied, bewildered. "Do you think you can get us a tow truck?"

I climbed onto the embankment with Larry and his sons, and heard the chorus of wails, yelps, and airhorns from the police cars, ambulances, and fire engine descending upon the scene from both north and south. I looked at the man and smiled. "That's not all you're getting."

"Oh my God," the man said, just now seeing the flashing lights approaching.

"I guess I'd better take the chopper off standby," Will said, keying the microphone of his radio to cancel the helicopter and as many of the emergency vehicles as possible.

Although he managed to call off the helicopter, Will was too late to prevent most of the other vehicles from responding. Within minutes two ambulances, a fire truck, and three police cars had arrived. As we stood on the embankment in the last light of the twilight, we could see a steady stream of flashing blue and green lights, some being switched off as we watched. Finally we made out the yellow strobes of the You-Maul-We-Haul tow truck.

As Larry started toward the tow truck, his nine-year-old son Art tugged at my sleeve. I looked down and saw the multicolored emergency lights reflected in his wide, amazed eyes.

"Wow," he said. "Does this always happen when a car gets stuck in the mud?"

"Not usually, son," I replied, shaking my head in disbelief. "Not usually."

EMTs often turn off their emotions when dealing with patients because they find dealing with the pain and tragedy that are integral parts of emergency medical work too difficult. Most maintain their ability to feel and relate to patients without sacrificing their ability to function effectively. Some don't.

For me, one of the frustrations of emergency medical work is the fleetingness of my relationships with patients. My contact with a patient typically lasts less than an hour, but may include almost the entire range of human emotions, from empathy and admiration to fear and anger.

On a currently popular TV program, the rescuers always become close friends with their patients. But for me the reality is that once I leave my patients at the hospital, I rarely see or hear from them again, and I seldom learn what became of them.

There have been some exceptions: the mother of the baby that Joan and I delivered in a stranded ambulance during an ice storm, who subsequently hired my daughter Davida as the child's baby-sitter. And Brad ...

I had just dropped Davida off at the mall and was approaching the parkway on Route 161 heading for home when the tones of my portable radio sounded. The tones were those used to set off the ambulance pagers in Davenport, the town just north of Prescott.

"Davenport police to the Ambulance Corps. A full crew is needed to respond to a reported PIAA on the parkway, one mile north of the town line. Car versus motorcycle."

That's just over the line, I thought. It will take DVAC some time to assemble a crew, and the parkway is almost five miles from DVAC headquarters. I'm only about two minutes away. I made a right turn onto the northbound entrance ramp of the parkway, reached for the plug of my green emergency light, then decided not to.

Because of rivalries and feelings of "turf" between neighboring ambulance corps and rescue squads, an EMT who "jumps" or "buffs" a call in a district not his or her own is not always welcome, particularly if he or she does not show proper deference to the authority of the agency in charge. These turf feelings are exacerbated by medical personnel with inflated egos, be they EMTs, paramedics, or even doctors who attempt to take over the scene and do not respect the authority of the local volunteers.

As an EMT instructor who had trained many of the DVAC volunteers, I didn't expect to encounter any problems, but since I was responding to a call that was not in my district, it would be prudent not to use my emergency light. It would be better if "I just happened to be driving by" and stopped to help. As I headed north on the parkway, I mused on the silliness of having to use such a ruse. Oh, well, I thought, egos are egos, whether they belong to doctors, emergency medical volunteers, or members of street gangs.

As I approached the scene of the accident, I saw a big highway maintenance truck in the left lane, its yellow lights flashing. In front of the truck was an orange-helmeted highway maintenance worker in his forties supporting a young man of about twenty, who was sitting and leaning against him. Next to them was a black 1000 cc Harley, lying on its side.

I pulled over onto the shoulder and, after carefully observing the scene and making sure that it was safe, I grabbed my crash kit and walked over to them.

"Hi. I'm Ed. I'm an emergency medical technician. What happened?"

"Hi, Ed. I'm Brad. Nice to meet you," the young man responded cheerfully. He looked completely calm and appeared to be uninjured, except for his left leg where his trousers were bloody. "I got cut off by a car and swerved into the divider. My leg got caught between my bike and the guardrail. Then I went down and the bike fell on top of me. This guy"—he nodded toward the highway worker—"pulled the bike off me and helped me sit up."

From the size of the highway worker, I figured that he could have lifted the heavy bike in one hand. It was too bad that he had helped Brad to a sitting position though. It's always dangerous to move an injured person.

"I can't believe it," Brad continued. "The car that cut me off never even stopped. While I was pinned under the bike, cars kept driving by, ignoring me. One car slowed down, the driver looked directly at me, then drove away. If this guy hadn't come and pulled the bike off of me, I would still be pinned under it."

The highway worker looked embarrassed at all the attention. "I was working down the road," he explained, "and saw the brake lights of the cars. I knew something was wrong, so I got in the truck and drove up."

"I'm going to check you out, Brad. Okay?" I asked.

"Okay," Brad said.

"Where are you hurt?"

"Just my left leg."

"Do you have pain anywhere else?"

"No, just my leg."

"Are you having any trouble breathing?"

"No. No trouble at all."

"Brad, I don't want you to move while I examine you. Let me do all the work. That's what I get paid the big bucks for. Okay?"

"Yeah, sure. Volunteers. Big bucks."

I opened Brad's shirt and examined his chest. It appeared to be uninjured and he was breathing normally. I reached behind him and palpated every part of his head, neck, and spine that I could reach without moving him. "Let me know if anything hurts when I touch it," I said. There was no deformity or point tenderness in his spinal column. I held out my hands to him. "I want you to squeeze both of my hands with yours, Brad." He grasped my hands and squeezed with equal pressure. "Can you move your uninjured leg?" I asked. Brad moved his right foot. So far, so good, I thought. No indication of spinal injury, although that could not be completely ruled out without an X ray.

"I'm going to check your left leg," I told Brad. "But I'll have to cut your pants."

"Go for it. They're all bloody anyway," he replied cheerfully.

"You would be better off lying down," I suggested. Since he had already moved and we would have to lay him down to transport him anyway, I wanted to take the standard precautions against shock.

"No. I want to see what you are doing," he replied.

Since he didn't seem to be severely injured, I didn't insist.

Using my shears, I cut open his left trouser leg from the bottom all the way up to his hip. Brad's calmness and cheerfulness had not prepared me for what I found. I tried not to let Brad hear the shock in my voice, but he was watching me. I couldn't lie to him even if I wanted to. And I didn't want to.

"Your leg's pretty messed up," I told him in a voice that must have been far from steady.

"Yeah, I could have told you that before you looked," he replied.

Brad's leg had evidently been crushed between his motorcycle and the steel guardrail and again when the heavy bike had fallen on him. He had multiple fractures of the bones of both his upper and lower leg. The sharp bone ends had penetrated his skin in a number of places, and white bone fragments could be seen through the open wounds. It was the worst leg injury I had ever seen on a living person.

"Brad, I want you to lie down so that you don't go into shock," I ordered in my most authoritative tone of voice.

"No," he replied emphatically. "I want to watch what's happening."

A Davenport fire engine pulled up and a helmeted firefighter dressed in full turnout gear came over. "Hi, Ed," she said. "What do you need?"

I recognized Christine Blakely. She had been one of the best of my EMT students and was both a firefighter and a member of DVAC. "Give me a hand, Chris," I asked.

She pulled off her helmet and heavy jacket and knelt beside me. I could sense the effort it took for her to show nothing of the shock that I knew she must feel at the sight of the massive injury.

"Brad," I said, "we need to get your boot off. We'll

be as gentle as possible, but we may not be able to avoid moving your leg a little. It's gonna hurt like hell."

"Go ahead," Brad replied.

"Chris, try to slide his boot off. If you can't do it without moving his leg, we'll try the heavy shears."

I supported Brad's leg while Chris slowly eased his boot off, then, using the shears, cut off his sock. During the entire procedure, Brad watched with his teeth clenched. Occasionally he sucked in a breath and hissed at the pain.

With relief I observed that the skin color of his foot was normal. I pressed his big toe between my thumb and forefinger. "Brad. What toe am I touching?" I asked, watching the pink color rapidly returning to the toenail bed, which had turned white under the pressure of my fingers.

"My big toe," Brad answered.

Thank God, I thought. Good circulation and neurological function. Amazingly it appeared that the broken bone ends in Brad's leg hadn't cut any major arteries or nerves. Maybe there was a chance, however small, that his leg could be saved, and maybe not. The injuries seemed to be too severe.

The DVAC ambulance pulled up and Ben Cohen came over carrying a trauma kit.

"Hi, Ben. Are you crew chief?" I asked.

"Yeah. What have we got?"

"Multiple open tib-fib and femur fractures, but no apparent neurological or circulatory impairment in the injured leg. I've done complete primary and secondary surveys and everything else seems to be okay."

Ben turned to his two other crew members. "We'll need heavy trauma dressings, a full leg splint, a longboard, and spider straps."

As we started to dress the wounds and splint Brad's leg, I continued to talk to him. "We'll be as careful as we can, Brad, but we will have to move your leg a bit. It's going to hurt a lot."

Brad was still calm and cheerful. "Do what you have to do," he replied. He watched as we worked on his leg, still gritting his teeth against the pain and occasionally allowing a gentle moan to escape. We worked quickly and soon were ready to immobilize him on a longboard for transport to the hospital.

"I'm afraid you're going to have to lie down now," I told him. "We can't transport you sitting up, and we're going to have to truss you up like a turkey to protect your neck and back during transport, just as a precaution against spinal injury." We eased him down, strapped him to the board, immobilized his head, and loaded him into the ambulance.

Since I would not be accompanying Brad to the hospital, I jumped into the Davenport rig for a moment to wish him luck. He smiled and said, "All I want is for this day never to have happened. That's not too much to ask. Is it?"

"No, it isn't," I replied. "I wish I could give that to you. Good luck, Brad."

I jumped out of the ambulance, watched as it slowly drove off, then got in my car and went home.

It was early evening about six months later and I was stir-frying some chicken for dinner when the telephone rang. Oh, shit, I thought. Still frying with one hand, I picked up the phone, expecting one of the usual evening sales calls. They always start out "Hello, Mr. Herman. How are you this evening?"

"Yeah?" I growled, waiting for the sales pitch.

"Mr. Herman?"

"Speaking," I barked, ready to hang up the phone and go back to my cooking.

"Are you Ed Herman, the EMT?"

"Yeah," I said, now curious.

"Did you respond to a motorcycle accident on the parkway last summer?"

Now I was getting worried. This must be a lawyer.

Maybe I was going to be subpoenaed to testify about some accident. I thought back to last summer and remembered the motorcycle accident. I had often wondered how Brad had made out but had not been sure that I really wanted to know.

"Yes, I helped out at a motorcycle accident last summer. Who is this?"

"It's Brad Forrester, the guy who was on the bike. I recognized you when you were helping me. Before the accident, I worked as the tennis instructor at the Fairfax Fitness Club and I used to see you working out there. I've been getting out a bit lately, so I went over to the club and asked around to find out your last name. It took me a while but I finally found out who you were and looked you up in the phone book. I wanted to thank you for helping me."

For a few seconds I was too stunned to answer. I turned off the burner and sat down.

"Hello, are you there, Ed?"

"Yeah. It's great to hear from you, Brad," I answered. "But I must tell you that I'm in a state of shock. In twenty years of emergency medical work, no one has ever tracked me down to thank me."

We talked for quite a while. Brad told me that saving his leg had been touch-and-go for a while. But after many surgeries, he was still in one piece and was beginning to get around on crutches. He sounded as cheerful and upbeat as he had at the time of the accident.

"The doctors tell me that I may have most of my leg function back eventually, but I know that I'll have it all back by next summer." He sounded absolutely sure of himself. "I'm going back to the club to do strengthening work on my leg."

Over the next three months, I saw Brad frequently at the fitness club. Then, one day in early spring just as I was finishing a last set of bicep reps in the weight room, I saw Brad limping over to me, without crutches.

"Hey, Ed. Boy, am I glad to see you. I was hoping

that you would be here today. Today is my first day without crutches and you were there when it all began."

I shook hands with him, trying to swallow the lump in my throat.

As he limped off to begin his workout, Brad told me, "My doctor says I'll be able to start playing tennis again in three months."

Brad and I will probably never be "close friends," as in the TV series, but there will always be an emotional bond. And while Brad may find it hard to believe, he has given me at least as much as I ever gave him.

On some calls we are required to make split-second decisions. Most of the time we make the right ones.

It was a Sunday evening and one of the coldest nights of the winter, again. For the third night in a row, the weatherman had predicted record low temperatures, and it was already five below zero as Joan and I prepared to go to bed. Although we weren't on duty, we knew that there had been a big wedding for one of the younger members of the corps and that most of the under-thirty contingent had been invited. There was no duty crew and, since the wedding was quite a distance away, there wouldn't be many people around. Of course we would be available, just in case.

I prayed aloud as I laid out some warm clothes just in case. "Please, Fairfax, no calls tonight."

"We don't have to go," Joan said. "We're not on duty."

"Yeah," I said, "but you know we will."

"Probably. Let's just pray for no extrications," Joan added.

Extricating victims of automobile accidents under extremely cold conditions is difficult for an EMT. It's virtually impossible to do it the way it should be done. The cold hinders our ability to function well and at the same time makes it necessary for us to work faster, to prevent the patient from becoming hypothermic—a life-threatening condition.

"I wonder how they do it in places like Alaska or Minnesota," I mused, putting a sweater beside my heavy jacket.

"Heaven only knows. I'm happy we work here. This weather's bad enough for me."

As I climbed into bed, I said, "And let's hope that, if there is a call, someone else takes it."

It seemed as if I had just fallen asleep. A beeping noise was dragging me up from one of the deepest, warmest, most comfortable places I had ever been. When the beeping stopped, I opened my eyes and listened. "Fairfax Police to all home units. A full crew is needed for a PIAA on Route 42. Any available units, please call in." An auto accident. I glanced at the clock. It was two-thirty in the morning. I rolled over and pulled the blankets over my ears.

When the police paged a second time, Joan asked, "Wanna go?"

"Not really but what the hell." I nodded.

Joan called police headquarters while I, now fully awake, threw back the blanket, swung my legs over the side of the bed, and started pulling on my layers of heavy clothing. "Damn," I muttered, thinking about the snow. "I forgot. I have no boots. I'll have to wear my sneakers."

As Joan hung up the phone and leaped out of bed, she said, "We've got a car versus tree. Since we're closer we're going to the scene. They're still paging for a driver."

"Shit," I commented eloquently, thinking of my feet. "Why do we do these things? It's probably ten to fifteen below zero out there."

The night was crystal clear, with a bright moon shining on the snow that had fallen a couple of days earlier. As we raced out of the house and jumped into the car,

I could feel the moisture of my breath freezing on my upper lip and the inside of my nostrils. I depressed the clutch, turned the ignition key, and listened to the starting motor slowly groan as it tried to turn over the engine.

The engine reluctantly growled to life. The shift stick felt as if I were forcing it through glue as it ground into first gear. The car balked and seemed to be saying, "You want me to do what?" as I depressed the accelerator. I knew that accelerating and fast driving at this temperature were murdering my engine, but I felt I had no choice.

With green light flashing, we sped through Fairfax toward the southbound parkway, then toward Route 42. As we drove, we heard Bob Fiorella call in that he was leaving headquarters in 45–01.

We could see the wreckage as we pulled up to the scene. The car had crossed the road and plowed into a tree. The front end was demolished, the windshield shattered, and the driver-side door open. Shit, I thought, whoever was in that car is probably dead.

Merve Berkowitz's patrol car was parked on the opposite side of the road, just past the wrecked car. He had just finished setting out flares to direct traffic around the accident, and another police car was approaching just behind us.

Merve met us as we got out of my car. "I can't find anyone," he reported. "There's no one in or around the car."

"No one could have walked away from that," I said incredulously, indicating the still-steaming wreckage.

Stan Poritsky parked his patrol car and joined us. "There are skid marks that look like he spun out before the impact," he said.

"Maybe he was thrown out on the other side of the road," Merve suggested, waving his large flashlight. "Let's look over there."

There was an open field on the other side of the road,

and the moon on the snow was so bright that we didn't need extra light. The four of us separated, each exploring a slightly different area beside the road. Within a couple of minutes Joan called out, "Over here. I found him."

As my sneakers filled with snow, I mentally berated myself for not having my boots. I trudged over to where the man lay on his back in a small drift. "We'd better get him out of here fast," Joan said. "He's semiconscious, and his speech is slurred. He must be severely hypothermic."

"Yeah, maybe," I replied as I knelt beside him in the snow, feeling the cold seep through my pants. I got a whiff of alcohol from his breath and added, "But he's also drunk as a skunk. Let me just examine him for bleeding. There seems to be blood on the front of his pants."

I needed to know how much he was bleeding. And fast. Thinking that blood might have pooled under the man's body, I slid my latex-gloved hands through the snow between the man and the ground, then removed my hands and looked at them in the moonlight. They were wet and snowy, but clean of blood. I repeated the procedure along his lower back and legs. This time as I did so I could feel something warm and sticky all along his buttocks and thighs. I withdrew my hands and saw that they were covered with a dark substance.

"He's bleeding badly," I said. "But Joan's probably right. He's probably also hypothermic. We can't waste time and we can't remove his clothing to find the source of the bleeding. It seems to be only on the lower part of his body."

We heard the siren and saw the rig pull to a stop beside us. "Joan," I said, "I know it's not protocol, but let's get the MAST pants on him, just in case, before we longboard him."

Joan ran to the rig to fetch the MAST pants. If he

was shocky, we could inflate the pants both to control bleeding and to reduce the effects of the blood loss.

"BP?" Joan asked as she returned with the MAST and the trauma bag. Bob was right behind with a long backboard, the bag of cervical collars, and straps.

"He's wearing a down jacket. I can't cut it or we'll have feathers everywhere, and I don't want to move him enough to get at his arm. Let's just scoop and run. We can do everything else in the rig."

I saw two other cars approaching, each with a flashing green light on top. More members were responding. I recognized each of the cars. One was Pam Kovacs's, and the other belonged to Phil Ortiz.

Within five minutes we had applied the MAST and loaded the man into the ambulance. My hands were frozen and I had become aware that both my pants and my socks were heavy with melted snow. "Ed," Phil said, "you're soaked and you must be freezing."

"I am," I admitted.

"Pam, Bob and I can handle this," he said. "Why don't you and Joan go home and get yourself warm and dry."

I was never so grateful in my life. "Are you sure?"

"Go home," Pam said. "We'll take it from here."

I gave Pam and Phil what little information I had, then Joan and I climbed into my car and went back home. We slept soundly until we were awakened at 10 A.M. by the phone. At the sound of the ringing, I leaped out of bed and began throwing on my clothing.

"Relax, Ed," Joan yelled, "We're not on duty."

It was Pam Kovacs on the phone. She told Joan that, as the corps' first lieutenant, she wanted us to come down to headquarters at seven that evening for a little informal award ceremony. Totally puzzled, Joan told her that we would be there.

When we walked into FVAC headquarters that evening, a number of corps members were there. Each of them congratulated us on our brilliant "save." Their tone of voice was so strange that Joan and I were completely baffled. We had no idea what we had done to deserve an award, and no one would tell us. In fact, people appeared to be stifling a laugh whenever we asked.

As we sat down at the kitchen table, Pam handed me a plastic container filled with chocolate pudding—to a round of applause and riotous laughter.

"Okay," I said. "I give. What's up?"

"Well," Pam said, "it seems that the driver of the car last night was the owner of a local restaurant. He had driven down county to pick up some supplies that he needed for the next day. On his way home he had stopped at a watering hole and had gotten himself thoroughly sloshed."

"I gather that his blood alcohol was 1.9," Phil Ortiz said. Almost twice the legal limit.

"Anyway," Pam continued, "he had been driving home with a five-gallon bucket of chocolate pudding on the seat next to him when a deer ran out into the road. He lost control of the car, and as it spun he was thrown out into the snow, but not before the bucket had tipped over and covered his pants with chocolate pudding."

"Oh, God," I said. "Is that what I felt?"

Pam nodded. "I guess so. No blood, just pudding."

"Yeah," Phil continued, "as we drove to the hospital we checked his upper body for injury. Nothing. His pulse was strong and his breathing was good, but stinky. As we began to check his lower body, through the MAST, we started to smell something."

" 'Do you smell chocolate?' Phil asked me," Pam said, continuing the story. "The rest is history. He was completely uninjured and was not even particularly hypothermic. Just drunk. And pudding-ized."

"He's now in the slammer," Phil finished. "He had two previous DWIs so he's gone, I hope for a long time."

Joan and I have long since given up hope of ever living down the night we put MAST on a patient and rushed him into the ambulance for a case of *acute chocolate pudding*.

Short Subjects

The codes we use on the radio seem to many like a secret language. The ten-codes, as they are known, are used to simplify communication and avoid confusion—to those who know the secret, of course. Ten-codes vary in their use from department to department, but we've used them in this book as they are used in the Fairfax Volunteer Ambulance Corps.

Some of the codes are obvious or came into common use during the CB radio craze, as 10–4 did. Others we try to explain as we use them.

However, sometimes the use of the shorthand becomes more rather than less confusing. For example:

"45–01 to FPD."

"FPD on."

"We're 10–8, 10–17 from FGH. We'll be returning via the scene and making a 10–42 before returning to HQ."

"10–4, What's your 10–20?"

"Parkway and 10."

"10–4, 45–01. Give us a 10–49 when you get back to HQ."

"10–4, FPD. Our ETA back to HQ is about fifteen minutes. Can you give us the times for our PCR?"

"10–4. You were dispatched at 17:03. You were 10–17 at 17:05. You were 10–19 at 17:11. You were 10–21 to FGH at 17:26, out at FGH at 17:41 and you're 10–8, 10–17 at 17:55."

"Thanks FPD. 45–01 clear."

"FPD clear."

* * *

Here's the line-by-line translation.

"Fairfax ambulance unit number 45–01 to the Fairfax Police Department."

"This is the Fairfax Police Department. Proceed with your transmission."

"We are back in service, available for another call, and returning to headquarters from the Fairfax General Hospital and Health Services Center. We will be returning by way of the scene of the accident (probably to drop off a member who responded directly to the scene in his own vehicle) and stopping for gasoline before returning to our headquarters."

"We understand. What is your present location?"

"We are now at the intersection of the parkway and Route 10."

"All right, Fairfax Ambulance Unit 45–01. Call us by telephone when you get back to your base."

"We hear you, Fairfax Police Department. We'll be at our headquarters in about fifteen minutes. Can you give us the times that we need to complete filling out our prehospital care report?"

"Certainly. You were dispatched to the accident at 5:03 P.M. (We use a twenty-four-hour clock for times on our reports.) You were en route to the accident at 5:05 P.M. You arrived at the scene of the accident at 5:11 P.M. You were en route to the Fairfax General Hospital and Health Services Center at 5:26 P.M., out at the hospital delivering your patient at 5:41, and you are in service and available by radio at 5:55 P.M."

"Thank you, Fairfax Police Department. Fairfax Ambulance unit number 45–01 has completed its radio transmission."

"You're very welcome. The Fairfax Police Department has now completed its radio transmission, and anyone else authorized to use this frequency may now do so."

Got it?

Chapter 7

As EMTs we try to keep ourselves from spending some of our soul on every call. But sometimes we get involved in spite of ourselves.

Meranda Diamond and her family had moved to Fairfax in the summer before her junior year and in September she began attending Mrs. Travis's homeroom at Fairfax High School. Meranda was a lovely sixteen-year-old with short curly blond hair, soft blue eyes, and a figure that made every boy in the school dream of hot dates and making out.

She soon began to see a lot of Gary Walsh, a senior and a member of the basketball team. Although he wasn't much to look at, he had a great sense of humor and a soft singing voice. Before they actually dated, they spent considerable time sitting together in the cafeteria where they discovered that they shared a love for old musicals.

On their first date, they went to a special showing of *Carousel* and, on the drive home, Gary sang each of the songs for an enthralled Meranda. They saw one another at least once every weekend for the next month, and each time their date ended with a hot make-out session in Gary's car.

"I can't go all the way with you," Meranda said over and over. "I mean, I never have. My parents. They trust me. I can't." But she knew she wanted to more than anything, and she knew that eventually she and Gary would make love.

Finally, one evening, Meranda's parents and both of her brothers were out for the evening. Gary came over and, as Meranda got two Cokes and a bowl of chips from the kitchen, she knew that that evening they would finally go all the way. For two hours they watched TV and kissed and touched. At ten o'clock, they went down to Meranda's room, a private space next to the seldom-used family room. Although it had once been part of the garage, Meranda had made her room warm and intimate.

Meranda wasn't surprised that there was pain, but she hadn't expected it to last. In all the romance novels she had read there was a little discomfort, then the pleasure took over. She waited, but it didn't happen. She knew it wasn't Gary's fault and she didn't want him to know that she wasn't enjoying what they were doing, so she lay silently and bit the inside of her lip so she didn't cry out.

She waited a little while after Gary climaxed, then said, "That was wonderful, Gary, but you'd better go. My parents will be home soon."

"You're not angry with me, are you?"

"Of course not, silly," she said, running her fingers through his hair. The pain was intense but she kept her breathing even. "But really, I don't want my parents to find us in here."

"I love you, Meranda."

"And I love you too, darling."

Suddenly they heard a car drive up the driveway. "Please," Meranda whispered. "Get going. I'll see you at school tomorrow."

Gary dressed quickly and kissed Meranda on her open mouth. As he heard her parents come through the front entrance, Gary slipped out the patio door.

For an hour, Meranda lay in bed waiting for the pain to subside. She felt what she assumed to be semen trickle from her body. Yuck, she thought. Now I know what they mean when they talk about sleeping in the wet spot.

After about an hour, Meranda had to go to the bathroom, partly because she had to pee and partly to clean herself up so she could say good night to her parents. It wouldn't do for them to get curious and come into her room. She stood up, felt woozy, and clutched at her bed's footboard to steady herself. God, she said to herself, if I'd known how bad this was going to be I might have waited a little longer. She pictured Gary. He's so sweet, she thought, and I do love him.

As she started toward her bathroom, she glanced at the bed. There, in the center, was a pool of blood. "Oh, God," she said. "That's not what they say in the books. A few drops, that's what's supposed to happen. What's wrong?" She struggled to the bathroom and sat on the toilet.

It was as if she had her period, but even heavier than her worst days. And, as she moved, there was intense pain, low in her belly. "I'm not due for another week," she said aloud. She thought about calling her mother, but what would she tell her? As she sat on the john she pictured her mother's face. "Sure," she said aloud. "I can just see this. Hey, Mom, I had sex with Gary for the first time and now I'm bleeding." Sure. Right.

She grabbed a heavy bath towel and a maxi-pad and slowly made her way back to bed. She covered the blood on the sheets with the towel, pulled a pair of underpants from her drawer, and pressed the maxi-pad onto the crotch. She hiked the panties up and, since she was very cold, she added a pair of sweat pants, a sweat shirt, and a pair of heavy socks. Exhausted, she dropped onto the mattress.

For what seemed like forever, she waited for the pain and bleeding to subside, but at about two in the morning she knew something was really wrong. Weak, shaking, and sweaty, but still not wanting to explain her predicament to her parents, she picked the phone up from beside her bed and dialed 911.

"Fairfax Police," the voice said. "What is your emergency?"

"I think I need an ambulance. I'm feeling terrible."

"What's the problem?"

"I hurt. And I'm sick. Send someone." She started to cry.

"Okay. Calm down. I'll dispatch an ambulance. According to my computer, you're at the Diamond residence. 479 Oak Hill. Is that right?"

Meranda caught her breath. "Yes. But they mustn't wake my parents. Tell them no siren, and tell them to come in the back, through the patio door."

"All right, they'll be there in just a few minutes. And your name is?"

"No siren. They mustn't wake my parents." Meranda's hands shook as she dropped the phone back into its cradle.

"What's your name?" The phone was dead.

Mark Thomas was dispatching at police headquarters that night. He turned to Officer Stan Poritsky, who was on break. "Stan, head over to 479 Oak Hill. I had what sounds like a kid on the phone. He or she sounds like she's drunk or sick. I'm dispatching FVAC."

"That's in Floral Court?"

"Right. Caller says to go in through the patio doors in the back."

"On my way," Stan said, walking quickly to the door.

As she lay on the bed with the phone beside her, Meranda thought, I've got to unlock the patio door. Weak, she stood up and felt blood gush down her leg, around her now-soaked maxi-pad. Hoping to sop up as much of the blood as possible, she pressed the pad tightly between her legs. Then she slowly walked to the door, supporting herself with one hand on the wall while the other held her lower abdomen.

Meranda didn't realize that she was leaving a trail of

bloody handprints on the paint. She turned on the family room light, unlocked the patio door, and half walked, half crawled back to her bed. Then she pulled the afghan over herself and dozed.

Ed and I got the call at home, dressed, and, knowing Bob Fiorella was bringing the rig, drove into the Floral Court complex. We parked just behind Stan Poritsky's car 308. Ed got his crash bag from the trunk and we walked up the driveway. We followed Stan to the back of the house and saw light coming out through a pair of large glass doors. "Caller seems to be a kid," Stan said, "and he said to come in through the back."

Together, the three of us crossed the patio and opened the sliding door. Immediately we saw the blood. "Shit," I muttered. "What the hell went on in here?"

"I better call for backup," Stan said. "You guys better wait outside."

"Not a chance. If someone called, the worst is probably over." Thinking back on that now, I was an idiot. "Hello," I called.

"In here," a small voice said.

"You alone?" Stan yelled.

"Yeah," the voice said.

We entered the bedroom and were assaulted by the metallic smell of fresh blood. I knelt beside the bed and looked into the terrified eyes of a teenage girl. Pulling on my gloves, I asked, "What's the problem?"

"I'm bleeding. It's not supposed to be like this but it is. And it hurts."

I stroked the girl's forehead, noticing that her skin was cold and clammy. "What hurts? What happened?"

"My belly. It hurts. It isn't supposed to hurt like this." She faded out.

I grabbed her wrist. Her pulse was weak and racing. In an effort to find the source of the blood, I pulled back the brightly colored afghan. "There's blood all over the bedding," I told Ed as I ran my hands over the girl's body, "but I've got no clue from where. Darling," I said, loudly to Meranda. "Wake up and talk to me. My name's Joan. What's yours?"

She opened her eyes. "Meranda. My belly. Help me."

"Okay, Meranda. We'll help you but we need to know what happened."

"Nothing. Nothing happened. Just hurts so much." Holding her lower abdomen, she slipped away again. Stan handed me a non-rebreather oxygen mask, attached to the tank that he had brought in from the trunk of his police car, and I put it over Meranda's face.

Suddenly we heard a shriek from the doorway. "What's going on here?" A woman in a bright red bathrobe stood wide-eyed. "Meranda, what's going on?"

"Your daughter called us," Stan said. "She seems to have been injured."

"Meranda. What happened? What did you do?"

"I'm fine, Mother," Meranda muttered. "Go back to bed."

"Don't be ridiculous. What's the matter?" She seemed to see the blood for the first time and screamed. "What's all this blood? Oh, God. Don't let her die!" She started to scream and cry.

Stan took the woman by the shoulders. "Calm down! You're not helping her by getting hysterical."

"What in the world's going on here?" a man asked as he descended the stairs.

While Stan dealt with Meranda's parents, I tried to ascertain what the girl's problem was. "I find no injury," I said to Ed, who was taking vitals.

Ed took the blood pressure cuff from the girl's arm. "BP's 100 over 70, pulse is too fast to get a good rate, respirations 24."

I helped her pull off her sweat pants and saw the blood soaking her underpants and the pad underneath. "Bleeding's vaginal," I said, turning to the mother. My first thought was that she had some complication of early pregnancy, possibly a ruptured ectopic one.

In an ectopic pregnancy, a fertilized embryo implants itself somewhere other than the uterus. If the fetus starts to develop in the fallopian tube, the narrow passageway that leads the egg from the ovary to the uterus, once the embryo reaches a certain size it breaks the tube and can cause the kind of extreme pain Meranda was experiencing. But there's not usually this much bleeding, I remembered from my training. This much loss of blood is life threatening, whatever its cause. I didn't need to know the details.

I covered Meranda with the afghan and turned my attention to her mother. "Mrs. Diamond," I said, having gotten the name from the dispatcher on the phone. "May I speak to you?"

"My baby's hurt!" she shrieked. "Can't you fix her? There's so much blood. She's bleeding so bad." She rushed to the bedside and started to lift her daughter and clutch her in an embrace.

Bob Fiorella called that he was on location, so Ed went back outside to get the stretcher. While I waited, I wanted to find out as much as I could. "Mrs. Diamond," I said loudly, knowing that I had to get her cooperation. "You have to calm down and back off if we're to help your daughter. I need your help and I need room to work."

Reluctantly Mrs. Diamond, still sobbing, stood up and moved to the head of the bed. When she quieted, I continued. "Your daughter's bleeding and we'll need you or your husband to come with us so the hospital can treat her. You need to calm down and help her. Now!" The woman seemed to slump as she nodded her head. "That's better. Has she ever had a severe period like this before?"

"No." She sobbed softly, grabbing her daughter's hand and clutching it to her breast. "She usually has cramps but not too bad."

"I'm sorry to ask this, Mrs. Diamond, but is your daughter sexually active? Could she be pregnant?"

"My daughter?" She stopped crying and glared at me. "How dare you! She's a good girl. She's never done anything like that."

Sorry I had mentioned anything, I turned back to Meranda. "Never done anything like that," Meranda said. "Never. Never."

"Meranda, it's all right," I said. "Just rest and let us take care of you." At that moment Bob Fiorella and Ed arrived with the stretcher. We quickly transferred the girl to it and covered her with two blankets.

"Who's coming with us?" I asked her parents.

"I'll go," Mrs. Diamond said, then turned to her husband. "Herb, you bring the car and meet us at the hospital."

We quickly got Meranda loaded into the ambulance and Ed and I climbed into the back with her. I lowered the stretcher so Meranda was lying flat and I raised her feet. As Mrs. Diamond started to climb into the back of the rig with her daughter, I said, "Please ride in the front with Bob, our driver. He'll give us all a quick, smooth ride to the hospital."

"I want to ride with my daughter. She needs me."

I felt a hand on my arm and saw Meranda's eyes on me. "Please no," she whispered.

"It's all right," I said softly.

Bob was trying to guide Mrs. Diamond to the passenger seat in the front of the rig, but she was yelling "I want to ride with my daughter! You have no right to keep me from my daughter."

I try to be nice to families of patients. I understand that they are under stress and may behave in ways that they wouldn't under normal circumstances. But this woman was trying my patience, and I was sure she was not doing her daughter any good either. "Please ride in the front," I said to the excited woman. "Our insurance company won't allow anyone in the back but the patients and members of the corps."

"But she needs me!" She shook off Bob's arm and

started to climb in the back. "You can't keep me ..."
Meranda started to sob.

"Mrs. Diamond," I said, "either you ride up front or
I'll ask Officer Poritsky to restrain you and you can ride
to the hospital with your husband." I could see the
woman considering her options, then she heaved a sigh
and stomped around to the passenger door of the rig.

"Thank you," Meranda whispered.

"Tell me what happened," I said before she slipped
out again. I could see her hesitate so I added, "We need
to know so we can help you. You know you're bleeding
and we need to know why. Could you be pregnant?"

"Not unless it happens instantly," she said softly,
through the oxygen mask. I could see her smile. "It was
really nice, except for the pain."

As the rig started for Fairfax Hospital, I suddenly understood. "Tonight was your first time," I said softly.
Meranda nodded. "It hurt when he penetrated?" She
nodded again. "Did you feel something tear?"

She pulled the mask away from her mouth and said,
"I didn't know what to expect. In the books I've read it
hurts, but only for a moment. This hurt for so long."

"Does it still hurt as badly as it did?"

"Maybe it's a little better."

"That's good." I gently placed the mask back over
her face. I didn't want her to be afraid of sex, so I
added, "It isn't supposed to hurt this much, and once
they get you fixed up, it won't hurt like this ever again.
Sex is a wonderful thing, especially when it's with
someone you love."

She smiled. "I think I understand."

"What's he like?"

"He's wonderful. He didn't know anything was
wrong."

"I'm sure he didn't. He wouldn't have left you if he
knew."

"Oh, no. He loves me. He wouldn't have left me
alone."

I held her hand and asked a few medical questions. Then we talked about love and men and sex. I took another set of vitals and saw that, although things weren't any better, they also weren't any worse.

"Are you going to tell my mother about what happened?" Meranda asked.

"I think you'd better," I answered. "She'll find out from the hospital one way or the other. It will come better from you."

"Would you tell her?" She hesitated. "Please? I can't do it. Not now."

Reluctantly I agreed. At the hospital, we got Meranda out of the rig and, as Ed and Bob wheeled her into the emergency area, I took her mother aside. "Mrs. Diamond, Meranda asked me to talk to you. Shall we sit down for a moment?"

I took Mrs. Diamond into a small room and we sat down. "Meranda had her first sexual experience this evening and something went wrong."

"She did *what*?" the woman shrieked.

"Listen to me, Mrs. Diamond. You have to decide how you want to handle this. If you make her life miserable you'll lose her. She'll do what her hormones tell her and she'll just stop talking to you altogether."

"But—"

"If you try to understand, maybe you can communicate with her, teach her about relationships. Understand this. Tonight she called the police rather than call you. I think you want her to be able to come to you with her problems."

For the first time since I met her, Mrs. Diamond was silent. I continued, "I think you'd better consider your reaction very carefully."

"Do you have any children?" she asked.

"I have two daughters but they are grown now. They live a thousand miles away."

"Do you talk to them often?"

"Once or twice a week," I answered. "And we can

talk about anything. That's a very special kind of relationship to have."

"Thanks for your advice. I'll think over everything. I certainly don't like it that she called the cops and not me."

I patted the woman's shoulder and, as she went to admitting to give the necessary information, I walked into the emergency area. "How is she?" I asked Ed.

"She seems to be okay. Nothing major that they are aware of yet. They're calling for a gynecologist, but Dr. Margolis said that she'll probably be fine and able to go home in a few days."

"That's good."

"How was your talk with her mother?"

"I think it went well. I hope that she'll understand how important it is for a girl like Meranda to know that she can go to her mother for help and advice."

I saw Meranda at the mall a few weeks later. She didn't recognize me and I didn't expect her to. But it pleased me that she looked happy and healthy and was walking arm in arm with a very tall young man in a Fairfax High School basketball team jacket.

Tom Markowitz had ridden with Fairfax Ambulance for seven years, starting when he was in his early forties. Tom was well liked, always quick with a joke. Frequently we found cartoons with silly added captions in our mailboxes, signed "The Midnight EMT."

Since Tom was a take-charge kind of person and a fine EMT, everyone wanted to ride with him. The local travel agency where he worked was open Tuesday through Saturday so he usually rode from noon to 6 P.M. on Mondays. When I began riding, I often rode that shift with him since, besides being a nice guy, he was a fine teacher.

I still remember one of the first calls I took after I got my EMT certification, a serious auto accident. Tom approached the car, then backed up. "You're crew chief on this one, Joan. How do you want to get this guy out?" After my initial hesitation, I dove right in, knowing that Tom was there to help me if I got into trouble or started to do something stupid. He made a few suggestions but let me make the decisions. The patient was well taken care of and I got my first dose of confidence.

About five years ago, Tom was diagnosed as having liver cancer. He continued to ride for a short time, but soon he became too involved in radiation treatments and chemotherapy to be available. All too quickly, much to our dismay, his condition deteriorated. Occasionally, as his illness progressed, his sister Anne, with whom he lived, called us and asked if we could round up a crew to transport Tom to the hospital for treatment. Members always volunteered to help.

It was just about a year after Tom stopped riding, and Ed and I were on duty as usual early one Sunday morning. We received a call from the police. "Joan, Tom Markowitz's sister just called. She says that he's having a great deal of trouble breathing and she needs you to pick him up and get him to Fairfax General. Bob Fiorella's coming from headquarters."

"We're on our way," I said, already dressing with the phone propped on my shoulder. "And tone out for one more person, just in case."

As I hung up, I looked at Ed. "It's Tom Markowitz," I told him. "He's having trouble breathing."

"Who's bringing the rig?"

"Bob. And you're crew chief tonight."

Ed sighed. Very seldom do we work on anyone we know personally. Doctors can select their patients and usually choose not to work on their own family and close friends. Personal feelings get in the way. But we had little choice. We could ask the police to tone out for some of the newer members who might not know Tom, I suppose, but that never occurred to either of us. We loved Tom and wanted him to know that people who loved him were taking care of him.

We sped to the scene and arrived before the ambulance. As Ed got his crash kit out of his car, Chuck Harding, the first Fairfax officer to arrive, called to us from the front door. "He's in real trouble. You better get in here fast."

We dashed into the house and found Tom lying on the bed, breathing noisily at only about one breath every ten seconds. "Too slow," I said to Ed who was already pulling a CPR mask from his crash kit. I took the mask and hooked up the oxygen inlet to the cylinder that every officer carries in his police car. I ran Chuck's oxygen wide open and used the mask to blow oxygenated air into Tom's lungs to assist his limited breathing. As I worked, Ed took vitals. "His pulse is 120 and thready and his BP is barely registering."

As I breathed for Tom I looked at him. Had I not known who he was, I wouldn't have recognized him. His round, open, cheerful face was now almost cadaverous. I mourned but continued ventilating.

As I heard the rig pull up in front of the house, I realized that Tom had stopped breathing. I shook my head at Ed who felt in Tom's skinny neck for a carotid pulse. "No pulse," he said.

"Oh, shit," I said softly. We faced a more difficult problem than usual. First, we were working on a friend. More important, however, we knew that he had always said that, when the time came, he didn't want any heroic measures. But that was then.

As EMTs, we have our protocols. We have a legal duty to act, to do CPR, unless there is a "do not resuscitate" order or "health proxy letter." In this case, without either, we had begun care and we were legally required to continue.

Ed keyed his radio. "45–22 to 45–01. Code 99. Bring in the CPR board and the defibrillator."

"No," screamed Anne, Tom's sister. "He doesn't want this."

"We have no choice," I said, breathing for Tom while Ed rhythmically compressed his chest.

"But he didn't want to be saved," she shrieked. "He wanted to die with dignity."

"Do you have a health proxy, a living will, anything?" Ed asked. Anne shook her head.

Normally, in a situation where the patient has made his wishes clear, we hope that the family is wise enough to resist the urge to call an ambulance when the patient stops breathing. In this case, however, Tom had stopped breathing after Anne called us.

Bob brought in the stretcher, with the oxygen duffel, the CPR board, and the defibrillator on it. "Oh, Lord," he said softly. "Do we have to do this?"

"We do," Ed said. "Do compression while I open the defibrillator."

Quickly Bob pulled out the BVM and hooked it to the oxygen I had been using. I then used it to force 100 percent oxygen into Tom's lungs. When Bob took over compressions, Ed opened a package of large shocking-electrode pads. He pressed one adhesive pad to Tom's chest, just below his right collarbone, and stuck the other to his left ribs.

"No," whispered Anne. "Don't do it. Let him go." She rushed over to me and tried to pull the bag-valve mask from my hands. "Please." She burst into tears.

I looked at Chuck for help. "Anne," he said, "please go inside and let Joan, Ed, and Bob do their job."

"But he didn't want this," she yelled through her tears. "Please stop."

Will McAndrews entered and helped Chuck to take Anne into the other room. Ed hooked up the leads and turned the machine on. "Everyone clear," he said as he pressed the "analyze" button and looked at the screen. "I see course v-fib."

I pressed my fingers against Tom's neck. "No pulse."

As the machine charged, Ed again yelled, "Everyone clear."

"Press to shock," the machine said. "Press to shock."

Ed looked around Tom's body, reassuring himself that no one was touching the patient. Ed pressed the button and Tom's body jerked. As he pressed the "analyze" button, I again felt for a pulse. "No pulse."

"We've got a rhythm on the screen," Ed said. I looked and saw what, in a healthy person, would be a normal sinus rhythm. Ed felt for a carotid pulse and found nothing. "EMD," we said simultaneously. Electromechanical dissociation, electrical activity in the heart that wasn't triggering any heartbeat. "Continue CPR," Ed said. Anne didn't have much to worry about. Tom wasn't going to make it.

Sam Middleton had arrived while we were defibrillating and now moved in to help us. Between cycles of CPR, Sam, Bob, Ed, and I transferred Tom to a long backboard and put the unit on the stretcher. Still doing CPR, we wheeled him to the rig.

As Bob drove to the hospital, Ed, Sam, and I continued CPR in silence. I wondered whether the others were also hearing Anne's voice yelling at us to stop what we were doing. When we got to Fairfax General, Ed reported everything that had happened to the doctor.

"He didn't want CPR?" Dr. Margolis asked.

"No," Ed said. "He didn't. But we had no choice."

"I know you didn't," Dr. Margolis said. He gave only one or two drugs, then "called the code."

At the wake, Anne came over to us. "I'm sorry for the way I behaved."

I wrapped my arms around her. "We all loved him and we knew what he would have wanted. But . . ."

"I know," she whispered. Ed joined us and we cried.

It has been several years since that night and I still feel badly that we had to punish Tom's body and cause his sister added agony. Fortunately, public awareness of the problems associated with "death with dignity" is increasing. We still, however, get put in this position all too often. And with nothing in writing, we still have no choice.

Since I take more calls than any of the FVAC volunteers, I've had more than the usual number of saves in my nine years with Fairfax. Although it happened more than seven years ago, this one still makes me feel wonderful and still puzzles me as well.

My radio squawked. "Fairfax Police to the ambulance corps. We have a report of an unconscious man at 342 Poppy."

"We need one more member," a voice said over the radio from headquarters.

"10–4. Want me to page out?"

The address was only three blocks from my house so I keyed my portable radio as I ran toward my car. "45–24 to Fairfax police. No need to page. I'll respond to the scene."

"10–4, Joan." I responded to so many day calls that, even then, many of the police dispatchers knew me. "The rig is on the road already with a driver and another EMT."

I opened the sun roof of my car and put my green light out the opening. As I drove the three blocks I ticked off the possibilities. Stroke, heart attack, diabetic emergency.

Pulling up to the small frame house, I saw several young men standing at the end of the driveway, waving their arms and yelling "Right here! He's on the side porch. Hurry up!"

I pulled to a stop and two men all but dragged me out of my car. "Hurry up, lady! I think he's dead."

"Let me get my crash kit," I said as I snatched a CPR mask and a pair of latex gloves from the glove compartment of my car. EMTs are the only people I know who actually keep gloves in their glove compartment.

"We'll get it. Just help him."

While one young man led me toward the side of the house, I tossed my keys to another and said, "In the trunk. The red metal tool box." I pulled on my gloves as I followed the other two around to the side of the house and onto the porch.

There I found a man, probably in his early twenties, lying spread-eagled on the wooden deck, unconscious. His lips and the skin on his face were bluish. I felt for a pulse as I listened for signs of breathing. "No breathing," I said automatically. As I pulled his shirt open, I asked, "Anybody know what happened?"

There were about fifteen people standing around, each giving a different story. "He fell off the porch." "He choked on a hot dog." "He just passed out." "We did some drugs." Without reliable information, I just had to do CPR, transport, and hope that the ER staff could help him.

I fitted the mask over the young man's mouth and nose and tried to give a breath. No air went in. His chest didn't rise. I tried again and still nothing happened. Retilting his head in an attempt to make a better airway, I breathed again. Still nothing.

Crawling around the man's body, I straddled his thighs. I placed my hands against his abdomen and gave about six abdominal thrusts to try to dislodge whatever was blocking his airway and preventing oxygen from getting into his lungs. I crawled back beside his head, opened his lips and swept his mouth, feeling for any foreign material. I felt nothing. I tried to give another breath. No success.

"Oh my God, he's dead," one of the bystanders cried.

"Do something! Do something," yelled another.

The young man arrived with my crash kit, but there was nothing in it that I needed. I motioned for him to put the box down and told him to wait at the end of the driveway for the ambulance.

Thrusts, sweep, breath. Suddenly, after several cycles, the man vomited, gasped, and began to breathe. I didn't see anything in the vomit that was substantial enough to have obstructed his airway, but I didn't need to know exactly what he had choked on. I just knew that as suddenly as he had stopped breathing, he had started again.

"Is he okay?" someone asked.

"Is he alive?"

I checked his pulse and watched for a moment as his chest rose and fell, his breathing labored but at a good rate. "He's breathing and he has a good, steady pulse," I answered. That was all I knew. "What's his name?" I asked.

"Andy," someone said. "Andy Carruthers."

"Andy," I said into his ear. "Can you hear me?" I got no response.

When the crew arrived, I put the patient on oxygen as I explained the situation. Andy moaned as we placed him on the stretcher and lifted him into the ambulance. By the time we got to the hospital, he was conscious and alert. He said that he had no idea what had happened and then would say nothing more.

We left Andy in the emergency room and, as we put new linen on the stretcher, several of his friends arrived, each loudly telling a different story to anyone who would listen. I don't think anyone even said thanks. I must admit I was disappointed. It was my first save and I guess I expected effusive gratitude.

We put the stretcher back into the rig and left the hospital. "Was he really not breathing?" one of my crew members asked.

"He was not breathing and very blue when I got there, although I'm not sure why. He vomited, then began breathing."

I still don't know exactly what happened or how I fixed it, but I do know that Andy's alive.

The call came in for a full crew to respond for a child not breathing. The address was a residence about one minute from my condo, so I called the police and let them know I would respond as the EMT. I dashed out of my house, still wearing an old sweatshirt and jeans.

As I pulled up in front of the two-story raised ranch, I saw a couple of police cars already on location. "Fairfax Police to all units responding to the child not breathing," the FVAC dispatcher said. "Officer at the scene says the child is conscious and breathing."

"10–4," I said into my portable radio. "45–24 is on location."

As I trotted up the front walk I could hear children screaming and loud voices. I opened the front door and was greeted by an unfamiliar woman's voice. "You two shut up. I can't hear a thing." The crying got louder.

"Hello," I called. I knew that uniforms often frighten children, so I opened my corps jacket so most of my grubby old Mickey Mouse sweatshirt showed.

"Up here." I recognized Merve Berkowitz's voice. He sounded thoroughly intimidated.

I climbed the half flight of stairs to the living room and was assaulted by the noise. Two children, a girl of about two and a boy of four, were screaming. A woman in her late twenties stood in the middle of the room with a squalling baby draped over one arm. Merve Berkowitz and Chuck Harding stood at the top of the stairs, their eyes wide.

"You children have to be quiet," the woman yelled. "I have to dress the baby so we can go to the hospital."

"What happened?" I yelled over the din.

The woman pointed to the two-year-old, sitting in the middle of the floor, shrieking. "Cheryl stopped breathing." She took a deep breath. "Her eyes rolled back in her head." She took anther deep breath. "She arched her back." Another breath. "She wasn't breathing!"

"She's certainly breathing now," Merve muttered.

A febrile seizure, I guessed. Young children often convulse during an illness, particularly when they run a high fever. The seizure isn't usually dangerous, but the child should be checked to be sure there isn't any underlying problem. In order to do that, however, I had to get some order.

"Ma'am. You're not helping your daughter. Try to calm down."

"Oh, Christ. She wasn't breathing. Oh, sweet Christ."

"She's doing fine now," I said calmly.

"Oh, Christ. It was so terrible."

"Ma'am, try to relax." All three children continued to wail so I took a deep breath and tried to calm everyone down. The police uniforms were a place to start. "Merve, Chuck, sit down and take your hats and jackets off." I was hoping their plain blue shirts would be less threatening than the uniform jackets. The two officers did so. "And when the rig arrives, ask the crew to wait outside," I continued. "We don't need any more chaos." Merve keyed his radio and I could hear him softly talk to his dispatcher.

I sat down on the floor to get closer to eye level with the children but I concentrated first on the mother. "Your name, ma'am?"

"Hargrove. Marian Hargrove.'

"Mrs. Hargrove, has your daughter been ill?"

"Yes. She's had the flu. Shut up!" she yelled at the two screaming tots while bouncing the baby on her shoulder.

"Is she feverish?" I asked.

"She won't let me take her temperature but she feels warm."

That's nice, I thought. Only two years old and already running her mother. I quickly realized that the mother was part of the problem, not part of the solution. "Ma'am. Why don't you go and take care of the baby? While you're gone I'll check out Cheryl."

"Are you sure she's okay?"

"She's obviously fine at the moment," I said, "but we should have a doctor at the emergency room see her. You take care of the baby, I'll take care of the other two."

"Bless you," she said, then disappeared up another half flight of stairs.

I looked at the older child. "What's your name?" I talked directly to him, so softly that he had to stop crying to hear me.

He quieted, stared into my eyes, level with his, then muttered, "Kyle."

"Well, Kyle, is that your sister?"

He nodded.

"Does she always cry like that?"

He nodded his head.

"It's hurting my ears," I said. "Yours too?"

Kyle nodded again.

"You know, Kyle," I continued, "she might be quieter if she had her favorite toy. Do you know what that might be?"

"She has a Barney," he said, snuffling.

"Could you do me a favor and get him for me? She would like that." Kyle nodded and ran up the stairs.

"Cheryl?" The girl had stopped crying and stuffed her thumb into her mouth. I opened my arms wide. "Would you come over here?"

She scooted away from me on her bottom so I put my arms down. "Okay, you don't have to." I lay back on the carpet. "I'm just going to lie here until Kyle gets back with Barney." I looked at her, my head now lower than hers. "Does your tummy hurt?"

Cautiously she shook her head.

"I bet you have a pain in your head from crying. It sure got loud in here."

As she nodded, her thumb still firmly planted in her mouth, Kyle ran down the stairs with a foot-long, plush Barney doll. I held out my hand for the pet. "Is this your purple dinosaur?" I asked Cheryl as Kyle handed the toy to me.

Cheryl nodded, now scooting closer to me and Barney.

"Is he sick too?"

Cheryl nodded. I figured this might be a good tool to do an indirect exam, since I had to wait for the mother anyway. "Does he have a pain in his head?" I said, petting Barney on the head. Cheryl nodded. "Yeah, I bet he does. Just like you. Does anything else hurt?"

Cheryl edged closer, until she could touch the purple animal. She rubbed the front of his neck. "Oh," I said. "Does he have a sore throat?"

Cheryl nodded again. She took the dinosaur from me and hugged it in her free arm without removing her thumb from her mouth. I leaned over and felt the dinosaur's forehead. "He seems to have a fever."

Cheryl felt his head, then nodded. "Do you have one too?" I asked. She felt her own forehead and nodded yet again. "Can I feel too?" I reached out and felt the girl's forehead. She was indeed hot.

Mrs. Hargrove came down the stairs with the now-quiet baby. With her arrival, Cheryl began to cry again. "My neighbor's coming over to stay with Kyle and the baby," she said. "Then we can go."

"That's fine," I said. "I think this was just a fever seizure but she should be examined." I turned to Cheryl. "Don't cry, darling," I said. "You'll make Barney's head hurt." Cheryl patted Barney's head and quieted.

The front door rang and Mrs. Hargrove let another woman in. "It's okay," the woman said. "I'll stay with Kyle and Timmy as long as you need. You just get Cheryl well."

I was still lying on my back on the floor so, while the women were out of the area, I held my arms out to the little girl. "Would you and Barney like to come with me in my big white bus?" When I got no response I said, "It's like a school bus, but it's got some neat stuff inside. And maybe even a new friend for Barney."

"Is she going to get a shot?" Kyle asked gleefully.

"No shots from me or anyone else on my ambulance," I answered. Kyle looked disappointed and Cheryl smiled.

Cheryl stood up, slowly walked over, and sat on my stomach. I sat up and wrapped my arms around the tiny girl. "That's nice, Cheryl. Can I pick you up? You're a delicious armful."

Cheryl wrapped one arm around my neck and we stood up with Barney scrunched between us. As I held the little girl, I felt her blanket-sleepers. They were soaked from sweat, tears, and probably a wet diaper. "Mrs. Hargrove, do you have dry PJs for Cheryl? She's really drenched. And maybe a dry diaper as well."

Mrs. Hargrove handed the baby to her neighbor and went upstairs to fetch dry clothes for her daughter. I looked at the two officers, each sitting still as statues in a chair. "I think we're okay here," I told them. "Would you go outside and tell the rig what's going on? I don't need anything. Just tell them that we'll be out in a minute."

Mrs. Hargrove returned with dry clothes. I took them, wrapped my jacket around Cheryl, and we walked to the rig. I felt the little girl relax and I was pretty sure that she had fallen asleep so I turned so Mrs. Hargrove could see her daughter's face. "She's fine and we'll take good care of her." I turned to Fred Stevens, who had arrived on the rig. "Nice and easy to Fairfax General. Our patient's doing just fine."

I climbed into the back with Heather Franks, the third member of the crew. Mrs. Hargrove climbed in behind us, and Heather sat her in the crew seat and showed her how to buckle the seat belt. While Fred drove to the hospital, Heather and I stripped the little girl, dried her off, and put her into a new diaper and clean sleepers. She didn't awaken. For curiosity, I pressed one of the strip-type thermometers we carry against Cheryl's forehead and took her temperature. It was 103 degrees.

"Some Tylenol and I think she'll be just fine," I said to Heather and Mrs. Hargrove.

"I gather it was bedlam when you got there," Heather

said softly. "Merve was telling us. You're pretty good with kids."

"I guess. I just try to see what they're seeing. Two uniformed men looming over the children, looking grim. The size difference alone would be pretty impressive to me. It was pretty noisy."

Heather chuckled. "I gather that's the understatement of the century."

At the hospital, I gave the little girl to Rosemary Harper, the head nurse. "You have a few of your own, don't you, Rosemary?" I thought she had either four or five children.

"Not one this little anymore," she said, taking the still-sleeping girl from me. "My youngest is almost seven now. Where's her mother?"

"Outside, giving the receptionist some information," I said. "She was part of the problem when I arrived, so try to keep her calm. She has three kids under five and, from what I saw, they drive her crazy."

Rosemary smiled. "What else is new?"

As I finished my paperwork, Mrs. Hargrove walked up to me. "It's not usually this bad," she said, smiling ruefully. "My husband's been away on a business trip and first Kyle got sick, then Cheryl. It just hasn't been a good few weeks."

"That's all right," I said. "We all get to that point every now and then. I can remember wanting to hurl one or both of my children out of a second-story window on more than one occasion."

Mrs. Hargrove sighed. "You were so good with my kids. How old are your children?"

"Mine are all grown up," I answered. "One's almost twenty-eight and one's thirty. They both live a thousand miles away."

"Thanks again."

"No problem," I said, hoping that she was now as calm as she appeared. Oh, well, I told myself with a sigh. It's not my problem anymore.

Short Subjects

Auto accidents frequently result in unusual situations.

One afternoon Ed and I stopped at the scene of an auto accident, which had resulted in a spectacular car fire. Neither of us had any intention of crawling through the flames, into the car. As a gust of wind blew the smoke in the other direction, we saw that two very brave young men had already dragged the driver from the vehicle. They put him down on the ground about ten feet from the car, which was now fully engulfed.

As Ed ran over to see about the people in the other car in the accident, I stood about fifty feet away from the burning car. "Could you move him over here?" I called to the two young men. "In case there's any explosion we need to have the patient as far from the car as possible."

The two men carried the injured driver to me and I did a full body survey. I found that he had a closed head injury, a broken leg, and possible internal injuries. His pulse was weak and his breathing shallow and rapid.

As Ed arrived back from ascertaining that there were no injuries in the other car, the local ambulance arrived and took over care.

I don't do fires. Ever.

We had immobilized the victim of a PIAA, had him strapped to a backboard, and were carrying him toward the stretcher. As occasionally happens, the man became acutely nauseous and we had to tip the man-board package sideways so he could vomit without choking. We lifted the man into the rig and, in case he had to vomit again, we foolishly decided not to strap him to the stretcher.

Since it was 2 A.M. and the man was in serious condition, the driver exceeded the speed limits on the deserted back roads. Ed sat on the jump seat at the patient's head and I sat on the crew seat at the patient's side. As we rounded a sharp bend the driver saw a deer standing on the road and slammed the brakes.

The rig stopped. The gurney stopped. Ed and I stopped. The patient-board combination slid upward across the gurney and almost cut Ed in half. Although he didn't break any ribs, he had a horizontal, blue-black stripe across his ribs for weeks.

And sometimes we make the mistake of believing our dispatch information.

Like the call for a possible stroke, which turned out to be a broken hip. That's sort of the same, I thought, as I began to immobilize the woman's leg. Each only affects one side of the body.

We were dispatched to a local nursing home for a woman with difficulty breathing. When I arrived, a ditzy aide was sitting on the bed next to an elderly woman who was propped up on four pillows. I checked her and found that she was having such difficulty breathing that she had stopped. As I got the woman onto the floor, I asked the aide, "How long ago did she stop breathing?"

"I don't really know," she said. "I think I heard her breathe a minute or two ago."

I shook my head and began CPR. The woman didn't make it.

Chapter 8

Some calls stand out in my mind, not because of the nature of the call as much as because of the people involved. Although Joan and I teach that there's no sex in first aid, occasionally we do get into awkward situations.

Sandy O'Connor Fernandez was a twenty-five-year-old, attractive young mother. Her long black hair, dusky skin, and high cheekbones intrigued men, and she could have had her choice from among many suitors, but she had married Nando, her childhood sweetheart. Now Nando and their three-month-old son Juan were the lights of her life.

Sandy really didn't like to take Juan into the supermarket, but she didn't have anyone with whom to leave him. So she planted the baby carrier-car seat in a shopping cart and wheeled it up and down the food aisles.

As she took a squeeze-bottle of mustard from an upper shelf, Sandy noticed an elderly woman trying to pull a glass bottle of pickles from the bottom of a stack. I wonder what's so special about that particular jar, Sandy thought. As she wheeled past, the woman jerked out the bottom bottle and the whole pile of large, heavy glass jars crashed to the floor.

Sandy felt her feet slip out from under her. Although her instinct was to hold onto the shopping cart handle and keep herself from falling, a stronger urge made her let go so that she wouldn't pull the baby over. She ex-

157

tended her arms to break her fall and screamed as she
felt the broken glass cut into her hands and the acidic
pickle juice burn her open wounds.

"Fairfax Police to Fairfax Ambulance." The radio beside me on the seat awoke as I drove toward the center
of Fairfax. "An ambulance is needed for severe lacerations reported at the A&P in town."

"10–4, FPD. 45–01 will be responding for a subject
with severe lacerations at the A&P. Please tone out for
an attendant to meet us at the scene."

I was near Joan's condo, halfway between FVAC
headquarters and the supermarket. The ambulance
would be taking the same route. I could continue driving to the scene, but there were three traffic lights ahead
and it was getting close to the evening rush hour. Traffic in town would be heavy so I picked up my radio and
keyed the mike.

"45–22 to Fairfax Police."

"Go ahead, 45–22."

"Negative on toning out for an EMT. I'm responding."

"10–4, 45–22."

I keyed the mike again as I made a right turn into a
parking lot. "45–22 to 45–01."

"01 on."

"I'm at the commuter parking lot near the high
school. Can you pick me up at the entrance?"

"10–4, Ed. Our approximate ETA to your location is
zero one."

As I parked my car in the lot, I mused on how we always say "approximate ETA." Estimated time of arrival
is already approximate. You can't approximate something that's already approximate. But then, the police always refer to VIN numbers: "Vehicle Identification
Number" numbers. Oh, well, I guess jargon doesn't
have to be good English.

I could already see the lights and hear the wail of the approaching ambulance as I sprinted toward the road. The ambulance stopped in front of me and I got into the back. Dave Hancock was driving and Phil Ortiz was riding shotgun. It was a good crew. Both Dave and Phil were first-rate EMTs, although Phil was still very young and, at that time, not yet approved for ambulance driving.

"Who's crew chief?" I yelled through the window to the cab.

"Phil," Dave yelled. Phil had started hanging out with the FVAC Youth Group before he was old enough to join and had taken every emergency medical course that had been available to him. Now he was a riding member of the corps and one of its best EMTs. But in many ways he was, at nineteen, still a kid, despite his 200-pound, six-foot-one-inch body. Although he looked like a football player, he tended to be shy and was as gentle as a proverbial lamb.

As the ambulance sped to the scene of the incident, I reached into a box next to the crew seat and withdrew a handful of latex gloves. "You guys need gloves?" I yelled to the front. "This sounds like a messy one."

"We've got," Phil yelled back.

I pulled the gloves on as we approached the front of the supermarket. I was glad to see Chuck Harding's patrol car there. As an EMT-police officer, he would have things under control.

"She's in the manager's office," an aproned employee told us.

As we entered the office, we saw a very attractive young woman sitting on a chair. Her left hand was swathed in gauze and Kling, and Chuck was just finishing bandaging her right. A howling baby lay in a carrier on the floor next to her.

I heard Phil behind me whisper appreciatively, "Wow."

"Hi, Chuck. What do you have?" I asked since Phil was hanging back.

"This is Sandy Fernandez," he replied. "She fell onto some broken pickle jars and cut her hands up pretty badly. The pickle juice was hurting her a lot so the store manager here washed it off with seltzer before I arrived."

"It was the nearest thing I could find," a red-faced heavyset man wearing an A&P name tag offered, "and I figured that bottled seltzer would be clean."

"It helped a lot," Sandy said, smiling at the older man. "The pain wasn't nearly as bad once the pickle juice was washed off."

"What about the baby?" Dave asked. "Is she all right?"

"She's a he," Sandy said. "He didn't fall at all. He's just crying because it's past his feeding time and he's hungry. Could someone get the baby bag from my car? It's the black Jeep with the red ribbon on the antenna about three rows back. The bag's on the front seat and the door's not locked."

"I'll get it," Dave said, realizing that things were well under control.

"I haven't had a chance to get a set of vitals," Chuck said. "I've been too busy bandaging her lacerations."

I introduced myself to Sandy. "I'm Ed, and this is Phil. That's Dave over there going out for your baby bag."

"And this is Juan," Sandy said, looking at the squalling infant. "He's usually not very temperamental, but he likes his meals to be on time."

I turned to Phil. "Why don't you take Sandy's vitals?"

"Sure," Phil said, remembering that he was supposed to be in charge. He was obviously delighted to be working on such an attractive patient.

While Phil obtained Sandy's blood pressure, pulse,

respiration rate, and pupil response, Chuck filled us in on the details of the accident and his findings.

"The cuts were extensive but there wasn't much bleeding. I pulled out a few fragments of glass but some are still in her hand. Fortunately, there doesn't seem to be any nerve damage and she has full mobility of her fingers. I think most of the pain was from the acid in the pickle juice."

Dave returned with the baby bag. "Okay, Sandy, here's the baby's stuff. Let's get you both into the ambulance and then you can feed junior. Can you walk to the ambulance?"

"Oh, sure. I'm okay except for the cuts on my hands."

I grinned as Phil elbowed everyone out of the way and helped Sandy into the ambulance. He elevated the back of the stretcher so Sandy could ride sitting up. As Dave got into the driver's seat, I placed the baby carrier on the bench next to Phil. I sat in the crew seat behind Sandy's head.

"Okay, Dave," I yelled to the front. "Take it code 2, nice and easy."

As we rolled out of the supermarket parking lot, Juan's howling increased in intensity. Sandy's bandaged hands were in her lap. She had not allowed us to immobilize them because she wanted to have some arm mobility for feeding her baby.

"I'm going to need you to help me feed Juan," she said to Phil. "This is a bit awkward."

"Oh, that's okay," he replied eagerly. "I can feed him myself if you like. I used to feed my sister's baby all the time."

"I don't think so," Sandy replied. "Well . . ."

"Sure I can," Phil insisted. "Is his bottle in the bag?"

"Well, you see, there is no bottle." She fumbled with the buttons on her blouse. "I, er, I don't seem to be able to unbutton my blouse with my hands all bandaged up."

It was all I could do not to laugh as I saw understanding dawn on Phil. His face turned beet red. "I can help, if you want," I said. "My wife nursed both of my daughters and I was perfectly comfortable with it."

Phil straightened his shoulders and decided to tough out the situation. "I'll help," he said.

"You sure?"

Phil took a deep breath. Nothing in EMT class prepares anyone for situations like this. "It's okay," he said. With the tips of his trembling fingers, trying desperately not to make skin contact, he undid Sandy's blouse.

"Would you pick Juan up and bring him to me?"

Phil picked up the screaming baby and settled him in his mother's arms. At last the howling stopped, replaced by a gentle sucking sound as Phil carefully examined the ceiling for cracks, loose bolts, or chipped paint.

Phil did not utter a single word for the rest of the trip to the hospital or back to headquarters. After we backed into the garage, the ambulance had not stopped rolling before Phil leaped out of the side door and ran into the crew room. I could hear him shout to someone, "Wait till I tell you what just happened. . . ."

I considered reminding him that all calls are confidential but then felt that it would be too much to ask of him not to share this experience with other corps members. I knew that Phil would never tell this or any other story in any way that would violate a patient's confidentiality. "God, she was so gorgeous."

Having worked closely with most of the Fairfax Police officers in emergency situations, Joan and I know them well. There is a sense of camaraderie and trust that comes from working with the law-enforcement people on whom we depend and who depend on us in stressful situations. And we often share intense emotional experiences: a save, or the loss of a life despite our best efforts.

Sometimes we share a laugh—as in the call for the woman who hit her own leg with a bowling ball; the attempted suicide who would not allow a medic to start an IV line because "I might get AIDS"; or the bloody but relatively uninjured teenagers who wandered around, slightly dazed, collecting parts of their wrecked car.

The Fairfax Police are especially wonderful to have with us in situations involving hostile patients.

It was 4 A.M. on a Sunday morning during the summer. The police dispatcher had asked us to respond for an assault victim in the parking lot of the Fairfax Diner. Bob Fiorella had been sleeping at headquarters and would be bringing the rig. Rubbing sleep from our eyes, Joan and I threw on our uniforms, jumped into the car, and drove to the diner's parking lot.

The area was almost deserted but it looked like the scene of a minor disaster. Beer bottles and broken glass littered the ground. "Looks like the kids have been hanging out here again," I commented.

"Your command of the obvious is overwhelming," Joan replied, grumpy over having been awakened in the middle of the night for what was probably the result of a fight between intoxicated teenagers.

The diner's parking lot was one of the local kids' favorite hangouts. The owners of the diner frequently called the police to run the kids out, but they always returned. We were used to hearing the police dispatch on our scanner: "Respond for disorderly youths at the Fairfax Diner." When the radio transmission wasn't clear it sounded like "disorderly ewes." Joan and I had a running joke about how the Fairfax Police often sent a patrol car to disperse disorderly sheep.

Patrol Officer Eileen Flynn's car 318 was parked in front of the diner's front entrance. As we approached, we could see a boy sitting on the bottom step, holding a cold pack against his eye. Eileen was talking to him and taking notes. Seeing us approach, she called out,

"Hi, Ed, Joan. This is Ken Williams. Ken seems to have gotten into an argument with a couple of other guys and they did a number on him."

Twenty-eight years old, just five-foot-one and very attractive, Eileen was one of the most easygoing, friendly, and effective cops in Fairfax. Joan and I had shared a number of difficult calls with her, and we knew her to be solid as a rock. We couldn't imagine her being hard-nosed, as we knew a cop sometimes had to be.

Ken sullenly allowed us to examine him. In addition to an eye that would be turning spectacular colors over the next few days, his upper lip was split and his nose was swollen and bleeding.

I saw the ambulance pull up and Bob get out and come over to us, carrying the trauma bag. "Let's get him into the rig," I suggested, "and then we can get a set of vitals and finish checking him out."

"I'm gonna stay far away from any patients tonight," Bob said. "I've got one hell of a cold and I don't want to share it with anyone. I'll drive."

"Sure," I said. "No problem. Joan and I can handle the situation in the back."

"Ken's only seventeen," Eileen advised us, "so the hospital will need a parent's permission to treat him. I'll contact them and have them call the emergency room."

Once we got the boy into the ambulance and sat him on the stretcher, I attempted to collect more information about his injuries. "Ken, were you hit just with fists or with other things?" I asked. If someone had done this with his fists, the assailant would probably need emergency room treatment for broken fingers. Most people don't realize that finger bones are more fragile than facial bones.

"Fuck you," the boy snarled. "None of your fuckin' business."

When Joan reached over to check his pulse, Ken

pushed her hand away violently. "Don't touch me, bitch, or I'll rearrange your face!"

"Joan, why don't you get Eileen before she leaves," I suggested.

Joan went out and in a couple of minutes the back doors of the ambulance flew open and Eileen climbed in. "I understand you've been giving these people a hard time," she calmly said to Ken. "Well, threatening people is against the law." Then, putting her face right up to Ken's, she yelled, "One more nasty word out of you and *your ass is mine. I'll bust you and you'll spend the night in jail. You got that?*" Joan and I were amazed at Eileen's transformation into a tough drill sergeant.

"Yes, ma'am," Ken replied meekly.

"I'm going to follow the ambulance to the hospital," she said to me. "You guys just pull over if you need me."

I had a hard time not destroying her performance with a grin as she climbed back out of the rig's rear doors.

"And you," Eileen barked over her shoulder at Ken. "You'd better make sure they don't need me."

Ken gave us no more trouble that evening.

One difficult situation we sometimes find ourselves in is when a seriously sick or injured patient refuses medical care. If the patient is an adult and in possession of all his faculties, we have no choice but to abide by his wishes, even though we know he may die. We use all our powers of persuasion and charm to convince him to let us help. Occasionally we even resort to calling the hospital to let a doctor inform the patient of the seriousness of the condition. But we can't force a sane and sober adult patient to accept our help. All we can do is ask him to sign an RMA, a "Refused Medical Attention" release stating that we offered to help, advised him of the possible consequences, and despite our efforts he refused medical care or transport.

I recall the evening we were dispatched to a residence on Franklin Street for a man with chest pain. The desk officer told us that his wife had dialed 911 over her husband's objections. When we arrived, the man was verbally abusive to us, insulted and berated his wife, and ordered us out of his house while his wife cowered in a corner of the room. Even the man's personal physician couldn't convince him to allow us to treat him. Angrily he signed our RMA, and we had it witnessed by his wife and the police officer at the scene.

We were called back forty-five minutes later, but by then he was in cardiac arrest. We did CPR but he was pronounced dead an hour after we got him to the hospital.

Sometimes, however, with the help of a police officer, we are able to "convince" a reluctant patient to accept our help.

Sylvia Feinstein, sixty-eight years old, was in a hurry to get home. She had finished her shopping at the supermarket and had stopped at the post office to get some stamps. She fidgeted with her pocketbook as she stood on line while the man in front of her explored every conceivable method of sending a small package to his son in California.

"Will it get there faster by priority mail?" he asked.

"Uh-huh," the bored clerk answered.

"But it will be cheaper by parcel post, right?"

"Yep."

"How much will it cost by first-class mail?"

Sylvia was becoming increasingly anxious. My husband will kill me, she thought. Sylvia's husband, Sol, liked to have his dinner on time, and Sylvia was going to be late. Suddenly the room started to spin and the air became so thick that it was hard to breathe. As the floor rushed up at her, Sylvia was aware of feeling pressure in her chest.

* * *

It was ten minutes before the end of our shift and I had just hung up the phone. The "extra cheese" would be ready in fifteen to twenty minutes, just in time for me to pick it up and take it over to Joan's. We were planning on spending a quiet evening at home, munching pizza and playing Boggle.

"Fairfax Police to Fairfax Ambulance."

Oh, well, I thought, so much for the pizza. Our quiet evening would be starting late, with cold pizza. I keyed the mike.

"FVAC on. Go ahead FPD."

"The ambulance is needed for a woman down at the Fairfax post office."

"10–4, Fairfax Police. 45–02 is responding to the post office for a woman down."

Dave Hancock jumped into the driver's seat and Stephanie DeMaritino rode shotgun. Dave drove out of the garage, then I pressed the button to lower the ambulance bay door and got into the back of the rig. Stephanie, who was crew chief, operated the siren, alternating from wail to hi-low with an occasional blast of the air horn as Dave carefully wove his way through rush-hour traffic.

As we approached the post office, I grabbed the oxygen tank and the trauma bag. "Woman down" could mean anything from a fainting spell to a cardiac arrest, so I had no idea what we would need.

When we entered the post office we saw a ghostly pale woman sitting in a chair with Officer Chuck Harding kneeling next to her taking her blood pressure. Chuck was one of the three police officers in Fairfax who had recently been certified as EMTs. "Hey, guys," he said as he saw us. "Would one of you take her blood pressure? I'm getting a crazy reading."

"What did you get?" Stephanie asked.

"I got 60 over 40. There must be something wrong with my equipment."

I took out the BP cuff and stethoscope from our

trauma bag and handed them to Stephanie. While she took the woman's blood pressure, I tried to find the radial pulse in her wrist. There was none. As Stephanie finished deflating the BP cuff she turned to Chuck. "I get only 55 over 40."

"I can't find a radial pulse," I reported.

Stephanie turned to the woman. "Ma'am, I'd like to get you lying down on the floor. Your blood pressure is kind of low."

Kind of low? I thought. I had never seen a person remain conscious with a systolic pressure of 55.

"I'm not lying down on no floor," the woman said, her voice strong and firm. "I'm going home."

"I don't think that's a good idea," Stephanie insisted. "How are you feeling now?"

"I feel like something's pressing in here—" She indicated her chest. "—but it's probably nothing but gas. I've been getting gas pains a lot for the last few days."

"Why don't you let us examine you?" Stephanie suggested.

"I don't need no examination. I've never been sick a day in my life and I ain't sick now. I'm going home. My husband'll murder me if his dinner is late."

"We can't let you go in the condition you're in, ma'am. You'll never make it to your car, much less home. And you'd be a danger to other people if you tried to drive." Stephanie was becoming increasingly frustrated. "You need to go to the hospital."

"What do you mean you can't let me go?" the woman replied angrily. "I know my rights. You can't stop me from leaving and you can't force me to go to no hospital."

"Ma'am," Stephanie said, "I don't want to frighten you, but you may be having a heart attack. Your life may be in danger."

"It's no heart attack. It's just gas and I'm going home," the woman snapped.

Stephanie looked at me and I shrugged. "There's not

much we can do. She seems to be lucid and she's right, we can't force her to go to the hospital. We'll have to have her sign an RMA and let her go."

Chuck had been watching us try to persuade the woman to accept medical treatment and transport to the hospital. Although he was a first-rate EMT, he always turned the patient over to us once we arrived and never interfered with our patient care. Now, however, Chuck intervened.

"Forget letting her go home," he said in his best police officer tone of voice. He turned to the woman. "I'm an EMT as well as a cop and I was the first EMT on the scene. You were unconscious when I arrived and your blood pressure is so low now that your brain can't possibly be getting enough oxygen for you to be thinking clearly. In my opinion you are incapable of making a rational decision." He glared at the woman. "You have two choices. You can let these people examine you and go to the hospital voluntarily or I'll place you in protective custody and force you to go. I'll handcuff you if I have to."

I wasn't sure whether he could do that, but he was making progress where we weren't.

Although Sylvia was dubious about the legality of Chuck's threat, she allowed herself to be transported to Fairfax General, where she remained for two weeks. As we all suspected, she had suffered an acute myocardial infarction—a heart attack.

There was no moon out and Lakeside Road was so dark and foggy that Chip Stevenson could hardly make out the edge of the road. As he steered his bicycle around one of the many curves in the road, he clung to the center line, which was about the only thing that he could see. He didn't want to ride too close to the edge of the road because he knew that, in some places, there was a sharp drop-off to the lake below.

Chip had been hanging out with his high school buddies at the mall, celebrating the beginning of the Thanksgiving break, and he was now on his way to his girlfriend Lynn's house. He had been working after school and saving up for a real set of wheels, but he still had a long way to go before he would be able to afford even a cheap car. His bicycle would have to do for now.

He had bought the stripped-down bike a month earlier for forty dollars and had vowed that he would put lights and reflectors on it one of these days. For now, however, he rode it as it was. It never occurred to Chip that, wearing his navy-blue denim jacket and jeans, he was almost invisible on the dark, foggy road.

Chip had just rounded the last curve before the turnoff to Lynn's house when a vehicle coming behind him lit up the road. He had started to move over toward the right when he heard the squeal of brakes and the blast of a horn. Suddenly he was flying through the air, out of the light and into darkness that was rushing to meet him.

Chip looked up. He was on the ground but he didn't know where he was or what had happened. In the glare of the headlights he could see a woman staring at him, her mouth moving. My brain must not be working right, he thought. She must be trying to tell me something, but I can't hear what she's saying. Someone's screaming so loud it's drowning out her voice.

Chip lay staring at the woman's mouth. He was aware only of the screaming and the unbearable pain in his head and chest. He had to get away from the noise and the pain. Chip got up and started running, but the screams followed him wherever he went.

The klaxon sounded just as we were about to turn on the TV to watch a rerun of one of the old *Emergency* TV programs. We tease new members that if they watch three hours of that program, they will become honorary

EMTs, and with eight hours of continuous viewing, they'll become paramedics.

"Fairfax Police to Fairfax Ambulance."

"Ambulance on. Go ahead Fairfax Police."

"We got a 911 call from a residence on Lakeside Road, about a quarter mile east of River Road. 10–2, car versus bicycle. Caller said it's serious."

"10–4, Fairfax Police, 45–01 is responding to Lakeside, a quarter mile east of River Road."

As we headed toward the scene, I heard Sam Middleton, the crew chief, get on the mike from the back of the rig. "Please put the helicopter on standby." Dave Hancock was in the back with him. With Steve Nesbitt who was driving, we had four EMTs on the crew. If the call was as bad as it sounded, all of us would be needed.

"10–4, 45–01. We'll contact county control."

About a minute later, as we approached Lakeside Road, the radio squawked. "Fairfax Police to 45–01."

"45–01 on," Sam answered.

"45–01, be advised that the chopper is unable to respond due to weather conditions. Also be advised that our officer at the scene requests you respond ASAP but with caution. There's heavy fog around the lake."

"10–4. We're responding as quickly as we can."

Steve and I glanced at each other in the fog-reflected light that dimly illuminated the cab and shrugged. "Respond with caution" means go slowly. "Respond ASAP" (as soon as possible) means "the situation is bad, move your ass." As the driver, Steve was stuck between the proverbial rock and hard place.

We could see the red glare through the fog before we actually saw the flares that lined the road. Guided by the eerie red glow, Steve steered the rig around the sharp curve and we emerged into a surreal scene. With the fog swirling around them, two police officers were trying to hold a six-foot, 180-pound boy who was struggling violently and shrieking nonstop. A woman was standing next to a car with a shattered windshield, watching. In the center of the road lay the twisted remains of a bicycle.

Steve pulled the ambulance over in front of the two police cars. As we got out, Stan Poritsky, one of the cops, yelled, "Get the stretcher over here!"

I ran to the back of the rig to give Dave a hand with the stretcher while Sam walked over to try to talk to the boy. "Where are you hurt?" he shouted over the boy's screams. But the boy would only shriek.

"We found him screaming like this and running around in circles," Stan shouted. "We were afraid he would hurt himself further, so we grabbed him. We have no idea where he's hurt."

It took all six of us to wrestle the boy against the long backboard that we had placed behind him. With Sam holding the boy's head, Dave fastened a cervical collar around his neck. Steve grabbed the board under one of the boy's arms and I grabbed the board on the other side.

With Dave and the two cops holding various limbs, we wrestled the board-and-boy combination onto the pavement, strapped him down, then lifted him onto the stretcher.

The boy's jacket was shredded, revealing numerous cuts and bruises on his face and arms. Sam sliced the boy's shirt open and found a large bruise on his chest. "Severe contusion," he muttered, "with several possibly broken ribs, but no evidence of sucking wound or flail chest."

The boy's rib cage was damaged, but there was nothing that we needed to do. I attempted to listen to his lung sounds with my stethoscope but could hear nothing over his shrieks.

As Steve struggled to get a set of vitals, Sam muttered, "No helmet, the asshole. And look at his clothes. He's fuckin' invisible."

I examined his head and found a large area of swelling on one side just behind his ear. With evidence of chest and head trauma, Sam decided that we had no time to spare. We tightened the straps to keep him from moving, immobilized his head, and placed an oxygen mask on his face. We headed for Fairfax General as fast as we could safely go in the dense fog.

By the time we reached the hospital, we were all unnerved by the boy's screams and were looking forward to transferring responsibility for his care to the emergency room staff. In the ER the boy remained combative, and we were asked to help restrain him while he was being examined by Dr. Margolis. It took all four of us along with two nurses to hold him down while a Foley catheter was inserted into his bladder to monitor his kidney activity.

"Sorry, guys," Dr. Margolis told us as he examined the boy. "I know this is hard on you, but this boy has a pneumothorax. I'm going to have to put in a chest tube, fast. I can't anesthetize him because of his head injuries, and he isn't going to like it at all. I'll need you to keep holding him."

I leaned over and yelled in the boy's ear. "Try to stop shrieking so we can help you. Try to calm down." He continued to scream and I stood up. "How can he keep screeching like that with a collapsed lung?"

"Amazing, isn't it?" the doctor replied.

While we held the struggling boy down, Dr. Margolis swabbed his chest with an iodine solution, made a small, deep incision, and inserted a tube. I felt momentarily nauseous as I watched the procedure, but knowing that I could not let go of the boy, I choked back the bile rising in my throat and held on. Whether from exhaustion or because he was able to breathe more easily, the boy began to calm down, and the hospital staff was soon able to control him without our help.

After we cleaned ourselves up and put clean linen on our stretcher, I glanced over Sam's shoulder. Chip

Stevenson was eighteen years old. At this rate, I wondered if he would ever reach nineteen.

We rode back to headquarters in silence, too emotionally and physically exhausted to even make small talk.

About four months later, Sam, Steve, and I had just come on duty to begin our first Tuesday evening shift together since Chip's accident. As with so many of our calls, we had never learned what had become of the young bicyclist. It's not that we couldn't have found out if we had inquired, and it's certainly not that we didn't want to know. But with bad calls, we are sometimes afraid to learn the outcome. We don't want to find out that our patient has died.

"Guess who I saw last night?" Sam shouted from the bedroom as he was changing into his uniform.

"Do you want to give us a clue?" Steve replied.

"Sure. It's a kid we all know and he's very stupid."

"That describes a lot of people I know," I said. "Why don't you narrow it down to just a few million?"

Sam came out of the bedroom, tucking his shirt into his pants and arranging the holster in which he kept his shears, penlight, and latex gloves. "I was driving down Route 29 in Davenport last night at about ten o'clock, when I saw a kid riding a bike right in front of me, in the middle of the road. No lights, no reflectors, no nothing. And he was wearing a dark jacket. I almost hit him. I passed him, then pulled over and flagged him down. Guess who it was?"

"You gotta be kidding," Steve and I said in unison.

"Nope," Sam replied. "It was Chip Stevenson, the kid we picked up a few months ago. I went bananas. 'Don't you ever learn,' I asked him. He told me to mind my own business and rode off down the middle of the road."

"Oh, well," I muttered, "I guess you can't win them all."

"Let's go watch an *Emergency* rerun," Sam sug-

gested. "I suddenly have a desire to see someone win at
least one."

We walked into the crew room, hoping that no call
would come in for the next hour.

TV and movie depictions of volunteer firefighters and
rescuers often show them dropping whatever they are
doing and rushing out to save lives whenever they
are summoned. But the reality of doing volunteer emergency work is really quite different.

For the past ten years I have been a single parent for
my two daughters and I have been working at home.
Being at home makes me a valuable volunteer for both
the Fairfax Volunteer Ambulance Corps and the Prescott
Rescue Squad, since I am one of the few people available to respond to emergency medical calls during the
day. However, FVAC averages about six calls a day
while Prescott Rescue responds to approximately four.

If I were to respond to every emergency call during
the weekday hours when most people are at work, I
wouldn't be able to earn a living, much less be a decent
parent to my kids. As it is, since I live in the Prescott
district, I responded to 233 Prescott Rescue calls last
year. I also took a substantial number of FVAC calls.
But I can't respond to them all. The fact is that very
few of our calls are actually life-or-death emergencies,
and many are for minor medical problems that do not
really require an ambulance, just transportation.

When I do respond, however, I am required to treat
any call as an emergency and to transport the patient to
the hospital, a one- to two-hour commitment, even if it
is something as minor as an inflamed hangnail. So
sometimes I must decide, based on the dispatch information, how important it is for me to respond.

Unfortunately, the dispatch information can be very
unreliable. Once I was dispatched for a head laceration,
only to find that the man had cut his head when he fell
after suffering a cardiac arrest. Or a reported head-on

personal injury automobile accident with serious injuries that turned out to be an RMA—the victim refused medical treatment, so no one was treated or transported.

One of the most frustrating dispatches is for an unknown medical emergency. You never know how serious the call might be.

Just like every other morning at this time, it had been impossible to concentrate on my writing for the past few minutes as I listened to the sounds of my daughter feverishly rushing to make the school bus. "Bye, Dad," she yelled as she pounded down the stairs and slammed the front door. I looked at my watch. Well, if her past performance was any indication, there was no point in trying to concentrate for another minute or two.

A few seconds later, I heard the front door open again. I held my head in my hands. Not again, I thought. This was the third day in a row she had missed the bus. Yesterday I had told her that if she missed the bus again she would have to walk to school. But it was cold and raining outside.

I know I spoil my kids, but what the hell. They're great girls and really do their best. They don't behave like spoiled brats, so I must be doing something right.

"Dad, would you drive me? It's raining pretty hard," she asked sheepishly, peering into my office.

I sighed and got up. "Let's go," I said wearily.

Ten minutes later the car was back in the driveway and I was back at the word processor, ready to begin again.

The beeper went off. "GRQ-325 Prescott to the rescue squad. A full crew is needed for a man feeling ill at 58 South Main Street. Please call in."

"I'll never get any work done today," I muttered. The May issue of the biotechnology newsletter that I write and publish was already late. It was due at the printer the next day. I tried to ignore the pager and get back to work.

"GRQ-325 Prescott to the rescue squad. An EMT is needed for a rescue call at 58 South Main Street. This is the second page. Please call in."

Now they only needed an EMT. That meant that a driver and an attendant had called in. But they couldn't respond without an EMT. I've got to get my work done, I thought. A man feeling ill could be an upset stomach. Besides, a Prescott medic would be responding.

"GRQ-325 Prescott to the Rescue Squad. An EMT is still needed for the rescue call. Please call in. This is the final page before mutual aid."

Shit, I thought, no other EMT is responding. And I can't let them call another ambulance corps because it will take much longer for them to get help to the patient. I punched the Prescott Rescue speed-dial button on my phone.

"Prescott Fire Department, Rizzo speaking."

"Hi, Andy, it's Ed Herman. I'll respond to the firehouse."

"Okay, Ed."

The ambulance was already waiting on the apron, its emergency lights flashing as I sprinted toward it. Sally Walsh was driving and Brenda Frost was riding shotgun. Brenda was a new EMT, still inexperienced but quite competent.

"Hi, Ed," Sally said. "You didn't need to rush. Some guy's feeling a little dizzy. It's probably going to be an RMA."

About three minutes later, we pulled up in front of 58 South Main Street, behind the Medic fly car and the Prescott Police patrol car.

As we walked up the driveway we could see that the garage door was open and people were inside. We walked into the garage and found Prescott paramedic Amy Chen taking the blood pressure of a short, muscular forty-five-year-old man who was sitting on the floor, leaning against the garage wall. His chest was bare and was hooked up to Amy's cardiac monitor. An oxygen mask covered his nose and mouth. The man was covered with sweat, and it was obvious that he had lost bowel control. But despite his condition, he was conscious, alert, and arguing with Amy vociferously. "I don't need all this fuss just because I got a little dizzy. Why don't you all go home?" He waved at us.

"Because you need our help." Amy deflated the blood pressure cuff, shaking her head slightly in an unconscious gesture, then turned to Sally and Brenda. "Get the stretcher in here right away."

"Oh, Lord. I don't need all this," the man protested.

While Sally, Brenda, and two other Prescott firefighters who had responded to the scene were getting the man on the stretcher, Amy turned to me and said, in a voice low enough that the patient could not hear her, "We've got to get him to the hospital as fast as possible. He collapsed and lost consciousness while working in his basement. He'd regained consciousness by the time I arrived, but he refuses to lie down."

The patient was sitting on the stretcher, arranging a pillow behind his back. "This is so silly," he said, settling against the pillows. "I'm really fine."

"Get him lying flat," Amy said.

Under protest, the man allowed Brenda to pull the pillow from behind his head and lower the back of the gurney. Amy peered at the heart monitor and said softly, "His pulse is 26, he has no recordable blood pressure, no radial pulse, and his EKG shows a third-degree heart block. He's having a massive heart attack but he doesn't have a clue. He may go into cardiac arrest at any minute. I want to get him into the rig and start a line as soon as possible." Twenty? I thought. The normal pulse rate is 60 to 80 beats per minute.

While the crew lifted the man into the ambulance, I turned to the man's wife. "What's his name?"

"Norm," she replied. "Norm Curtis."

"Has anything like this ever happened before?"

"No, never. He's hardly ever sick. He likes to do hard physical work. He doesn't handle sickness very well."

"Yeah, I can see that," I said.

"Will he be all right?" That's a question that's so hard to answer.

I tried to reassure the distraught woman. "Well, he's pretty sick right now, but we're doing everything possible to help him. The doctor at the hospital will be able to give you more information."

Once in the ambulance, Amy quickly began to assemble her equipment for starting an intravenous line. "Ed, would you purge a line please?"

I opened the plastic containers housing a bag of sterile saline and some connective tubing, removed the covers from the IV bag's port and the end of the tubing, then plugged the end of the tube into the port. Holding the bag up, I squeezed, forcing saline solution into the reservoir. Then I opened the valve on the tubing and allowed the saline to flow through, free of air bubbles. When the liquid started to come out of the end of the tube, I closed the valve.

"What's all that for?" Norm asked, seeing the intravenous equipment.

"I'm going to start a line so that we can give you some medicine to make you feel better," Amy replied.

"I feel okay now. I don't need any medicine." He glared at the setup I held. "And I don't need any of that shit." He struggled to sit up.

"Lie down," Amy insisted, pressing him down gently. "And you do need my medicine. Your heart is beating much too slowly and I need to give you a drug that will make it speed up. Now give me your arm."

Despite his protests, Norm extended his arm.

Amy quickly tied a constricting band around Norm's arm, then saying, "This will pinch a little," she inserted a needle into his vein.

While Amy and I started the IV on Norm's right arm, Brenda attempted to obtain a blood pressure reading on his left. As she allowed the BP cuff to deflate, she looked at Amy and shook her head. There was still no measurable blood pressure. I was amazed that Norm was still conscious with so little blood flowing to his brain.

"Okay, Sally," Amy shouted to our driver. "Let's go. Don't break your neck but don't stop to admire the scenery." Sally understood that this was a lights-and-siren situation but that Amy wanted as smooth a ride as possible and didn't want to alarm Norm.

As we headed toward Fairfax General, Amy injected a dose of atropine into the IV line. Then as we watched the heart monitor, we could see Norm's heart speed up. It seemed to stabilize at a more normal rate of 65 beats per minute. His blood pressure, however, was still too low to be measured.

"My arm hurts," Norm complained as we sped toward the hospital. "This thing's jabbing me."

While he continued to complain about his arm and the injustice of being taken to the hospital when he had just had a little dizzy spell, we began to relax a little. I could see, however, that Amy was continuously watching the EKG monitor.

"I'm going to complain about you people," Norm threatened. "You can't take me anywhere unless I let you. I don't need this. I could make you let me off right here if I wanted to."

Suddenly, without a word, Amy calmly made a fist with her right hand, raised it over Norm's body, and slammed it down onto the middle of his chest.

"Ow," he yelled, staring in amazement at the five-foot-three, ninety-eight-pound girl who had just punched him in the chest hard enough to knock his breath out.

Amy said nothing. She just calmly leaned back, keeping her eyes on the heart monitor.

I glanced at Brenda, who was sitting next to me on the crew bench. She appeared to be in a state of shock. I would be also, I thought, if I hadn't known why a medic would slug a patient who was in the midst of having a heart attack. Norm was extremely well be-haved for the rest of the trip, not wanting to further an-ger the crazy medic who was willing to beat up patients who complained too much.

At the hospital, after the emergency room staff had taken over Norm's care and we were finishing up our paperwork, I said to Amy, "That was amazing. I've never seen a precordial thump administered to a con-scious patient. What rhythm was he in?"

"V-fib," Amy replied.

"Oh, wow. Of course. That's why you punched him," Brenda said, obviously relieved to know that her col-league was not crazy. "Ventricular fibrillation is a fatal rhythm, isn't it? The heart won't pump enough blood to support life. Why didn't he stop breathing and col-lapse?"

"It all happened so fast that his body hadn't reacted to his change of rhythm yet," I explained. "Amy's thump restored the correct rhythm and his body never realized that he had actually been dead momentarily."

Brenda laughed. "Wow, Amy. I thought you were just pissed that he was giving you a hard time."

"Oh my God," Amy said, suddenly realizing the rea-son for Norm's change in behavior. "The man must have thought I was hitting him because of his griping. No wonder he was so good after that. I was just concen-trating on the monitor, afraid that he would code. And he did."

"I wonder if this qualifies as a save," I mused. It's quite a philosophical question. Does it count if you bring someone back from clinical death if the person never stopped talking and complaining while he was dead?

"I don't even want to think about it," Brenda said as we wheeled the stretcher out to the ambulance.

Short Subjects

The following story, about a man's amazing reaction to an accident, is from a letter we received from an emergency worker from Ohio.

I'd like to relate a rather light-hearted incident that happened to me. I, too, am a volunteer EMT with our local township fire department. My paid job is as a service technician for Sears Service. Part of my job is making in-the-home repairs.

One day I came to a railroad crossing and was the third vehicle back. The westbound train was a long and slow-moving one and, as soon as it was past, the first auto started across the double track.

As the second car started across I noticed the flashers and heard a train whistle. Looking west, I saw a fast-moving train, heading east. While I watched in horror, it struck the second car and pushed it down the track.

The car was finally pushed clear of the train and I was really apprehensive about checking the driver. But I knew what I had to do.

After the train had passed, I saw the car about one hundred feet down the tracks. Fenders, bumpers, chrome shards, and glass littered the track bed.

As I neared the vehicle, I saw that it had not been overturned, only spun around and, amazingly, the passenger compartment was still intact. I was surprised to discover that the seatbelted driver was apparently unhurt. While waiting for an ambulance to arrive, I stayed close and tried to maintain c-spine stabilization.

Other people came around, and one fellow who

knew the driver ran up and asked him how he felt. His reply made me feel a little more relieved: "I feel like I've been hit by a freight train."

He was holding his lips and a good chunk of his left
in his hands. "Oh God," Rita cried calmly, "I was
beaten to death by a firefighter..."

Chapter 9

The emergency services in every town work closely
with one another; therefore, we in the ambulance corps
know most of the police and firefighters. When a medical emergency happens involving one of our friends,
the situation becomes particularly difficult. The following story was told to us by several members of our local
services. We've combined the accounts into this story
and told it through the eyes of Fred Stevens, a longtime
Fairfax EMT.

It was the third day of an early-summer heat wave.
By four in the afternoon, the temperature had again
risen to over 100 degrees. Willy Monteleone had been
doing a little work in the yard and had just come inside
out of the broiling sun because he had begun to feel
dizzy. I guess I can't take the heat as well as I used to,
he thought. At forty-nine, Willy considered himself to
be in pretty good physical condition. A bit of a beer
belly, he thought as he patted his ample girth, but otherwise in good shape. He was about to relax with a cold
Bud when he heard the insistent beep of his fire pager.

"GCC-905 Fairfax Fire Department to all units. Additional manpower is needed for a brushfire near the
construction site on the parkway."

"Shit," Willy muttered, "what a day for a lousy
brushfire." He sighed, then put his beer down. "I guess
I ought to go. Lucky I haven't had any of this beer yet."
He wouldn't have dreamed of responding to a call
184

under the influence of alcohol. Willy heaved himself out of his easy chair and yelled, "Hon, I'm going to respond to that fire call."

"Sure, honey," Carol Monteleone, Willy's wife of twenty-two years, said. "Call me if you get a chance." Her husband had been a member of the Fairfax Fire Department since before they were married, and she had grown used to his sudden comings and goings. She mentally put her plans for an early dinner on hold, knowing that Willy would probably be gone for a couple of hours.

No longer dizzy, Willy lumbered out to his car, turned on his flashing blue light, and started toward the parkway.

As Willy drove up the long slope from Route 10 and pulled up next to several cars with blue lights on the top, he saw two pumpers with hoses stretched into a brushy area next to some large pieces of construction equipment. Off to one side, an FVAC rig sat, just in case it was needed.

"Hi, Willy," his friend and fellow firefighter Ken Stavitsky yelled. Ken was heading toward a large Styrofoam water barrel for a drink. "Small fire but a real pain in the ass. Just when we get it knocked down one place, it pops up somewhere else. Thanks for coming." Willy could see several firefighters joined by members of the highway construction crew using rakes, pitchforks, and small handaxes to clear the leaves and debris through and under which the fire had been moving.

Willy rummaged in his trunk and found his heavy turnout gear. "Fuckin' heat," he muttered. "I hope we're almost done." Reluctantly he pulled on the waterproof jacket, bunker pants, and heavy boots and put the black fire helmet on his head. As he walked toward the fire scene, someone pressed a rake into his hands. Joining the group already working, he and several others began to drag debris away from the latest flareup. *I could be* home, doing this in my yard, he thought. But, deep inside, he knew that he preferred to be where the action was.

Technically, all firefighters were supposed to wear turnout gear no matter how hot the weather, but after about a half an hour the chief allowed them to take off the heavy fire-protective coats and helmets. "Leave on the pants and boots to protect yourself from embers," he yelled as the exhausted and overheated firefighters removed their outer clothing.

As Willy took his gear off, he felt a bit dizzy again. Better get some water, he thought, dumping his gear beside his car. He grabbed a large cup of cold water from the cooler, then returned to his rake.

Ken hacked brush with a small ax beside Willy. "As if the heat isn't enough," Ken said, his words coming in little puffs, "Gloria says that the weather bureau issued an ozone alert. The air isn't fit to breathe."

"What the hell do they expect us to do," Willy muttered, standing and trying to rub the tightness out of his neck, "hold our breath till the fall?" Even though he was used to smoke after all his years of firefighting, he was having more trouble breathing than usual. It must be the fucking ozone, he thought.

Suddenly, as Willy was raking dead vines toward Tom Cavanaugh, who was hosing the area down, he fell forward beside his rake.

Ken saw him go down. "Willy, are you all right?"

Willy lay facedown, silent.

"Tom," Ken yelled, "looks like Willy fainted. Let's get him away from this heat."

Ken and Tom grabbed Willy under the arms and dragged him about twenty feet down the hill, away from the smoke and burning brush, to a sandy, dusty area where the construction workers usually parked. They turned Willy over onto his back. His face was blue and his open eyes stared sightlessly. His chest heaved as he drew one deep, shuddering breath.

"He's breathing," Tom said. "Is he okay?"

Ken, both a firefighter and an experienced EMT with FVAC, recognized Willy's breathing as agonal, the type of breathing that precedes death. Kneeling next to Willy, Ken placed his index and middle fingers against the side of his friend's neck. Feeling nothing, he moved his fingers around, trying to find a carotid pulse. Willy took another deep breath, exhaling with a loud sigh.

"Willy's down!" Tom yelled. "Somebody help!"

Other firefighters came running up, brown dust swirling around their feet. Gerry McCarthy, an assistant chief with CPR training, knelt in the dirt on the other side of Willy's head from Ken.

"Anything?" he asked watching Ken's fingers probe for a pulse.

"Nothing."

Ken removed his fingers from Willy's neck, balled his right hand into a fist, raised it above the center of Willy's chest, and slammed it down. He again placed his fingers against Willy's neck. Gerry looked at Ken hopefully.

"Nothing," Ken repeated as he tore Willy's shirt open and got into position to begin CPR compressions. "Get the VAC, stat," he said. Gerry tilted Willy's head back, pinched his nostrils together, and blew two full breaths into his mouth.

As Ken began to compress Willy's chest, Gerry turned to Mike DeVito, one of the younger firefighters. "Mike, get the ambulance people over here with the defibrillator, oxygen, and a BVM. And, Mike, call Prescott and have them dispatch their medic."

Fairfax Volunteer Ambulance Corps sends an ambulance to every "working" structure fire—that is, a fire in a house or similar building where firefighters are actually wetting down, chopping to gain access, moving gas and oil tanks, and the like. We are there to treat any victims of the original fire and to deal with firefighters who need oxygen, fluids, and, occasionally, burn or injury treatment.

Usually there is nothing to do, and many of us find fire standbys a complete bore. Luckily, some of our members enjoy watching the firefighters in action so, when the dispatcher pages out for a crew to stand by at a fire scene, people usually respond. That afternoon I had been hanging around corps headquarters and had found it hard not to volunteer when the chief called by phone and asked for a rig to stand by. "It's not a structure fire, and I don't expect any burns or injuries, but I'm worried about this heat."

So, unable to duck out the back door, Nick Abrams and I had "volunteered." By the time Willy went down, we had been sitting in the rig for over two hours with the engine running and the air-conditioner cranked up high. Usually we would be bombarded with requests for water, but the fire department had been wise enough to bring a large cooler and had been handing out water left and right.

"I wonder what they need us here for," I had muttered several times. I had even asked a chief about an hour earlier whether we could leave. "Someone might cut his foot off with one of those axes," he had said, "or step on a rake and knock himself out. So hang in there for a while longer. If you get another call, however, you can go."

When I saw Mike DeVito run up, I figured that we might have to treat a minor injury. But my heart began to pound when I saw how agitated he was. Since I know most of the firefighters, I took a deep breath, afraid to hear what the problem was and who was involved.

Nick opened his door as Mike ran toward us, waving wildly. "Firefighter's down," Mike screamed. "They're doing CPR."

"Who?" I yelled.

"Willy Monteleone. I think he's dead."

I knew Willy only by sight, and I knew I had to put any personal feelings out of my mind. Nick grabbed the megaduffel and headed toward the "man down" while I got the defibrillator and suction and sprinted through the dust and heat right behind.

I saw Gerry and Ken, both of whom I knew from other calls we had done together, doing CPR as Nick and I ran up with the equipment.

As Gerry and Ken started to back off and let us take over, Nick said calmly, "Just continue what you're doing while we get organized. You're doing fine."

I quickly attached the BVM to the oxygen tank, opened the tank valve, and turned the regulator setting to 15 liters per minute. I let the reservoir fill with oxygen, then handed the attached mask to Gerry, who was red-faced and puffing heavily. "You hold, I'll squeeze," I said. Gerry held the mask sealed over Willy's face and I squeezed the bag, forcing pure oxygen into Willy's lungs. As we worked, I watched as Ken continued to compress Willy's chest, forcing his heart to pump. He was obviously overheated and tiring rapidly.

"Let someone take over," I suggested as I watched the sweat pour down Ken's reddened face. "You must be bushed in this heat."

"I'm fine," Ken puffed.

"Never mind fine," I said, knowing that he would exhaust himself without realizing it, running on adrenaline as he was. "Mike," I said to a fireman I recognized from a recent CPR course I had taught, "take over compressions."

"No," Ken said, pushing Mike away. "I'll stay here."

"Ken—"

"I'm all right!"

I wasn't going to fight with him so I nodded. "Gerry, let Mike relieve you." Gerry, sensing that his action might encourage Ken to let someone else help, backed off and Mike took his place.

"Ken," Gerry said, "let me."

"Let me do this, damn it," Ken snapped, and Gerry backed off.

While we worked, Nick unzipped the case from the defibrillator and pulled out a pair of large, shocking-electrode pads. As I watched, he tore open the wrapping, pulled the leads out of the side of the defibrillator case, and attached the pads. He pulled off the backing and placed one sticky electrode against the skin under Willy's right collarbone and the other against his lower left ribs. He opened the top of the defibrillator and pushed the "on" button. "Stop CPR," he said loudly as he looked at the screen and pressed the "analyze" button. Puffing, Ken sat back on his haunches, pulled a large handkerchief from his pocket, and mopped his soaked face. "Stand clear," the machine intoned. "Stand clear."

"He's in v-fib," Nick said as the defibrillator began to whine, the pitch increasing as it was being charged by the battery. "Check his pulse."

I placed my fingers on Willy's neck. "Nothing," I said, shaking my head.

A mechanical voice came from the defibrillator. "Press to shock. Press to shock."

"Stand clear," Nick yelled. Everyone moved back.

Nick pressed the "shock" button and Willy's body convulsed as 200 joules of electricity coursed through it. As Willy's body relaxed, Nick pressed the "analyze" button again.

Since there was nothing for me to do at that moment, I looked around. Growing ranks of firefighters surrounded the inert body. I heard the words "It's Willy," whispered as more men arrived, abandoning their firefighting.

"Come on, guys," Gerry said softly, "get back to the fire and let the EMTs take care of Willy." A few grumbling firefighters returned to fighting the fire while others remained watching the battle for Willy's life. I looked at Ken and was glad to see that he had calmed down slightly.

As the machine began to whine again in preparation for a second shock, I felt for a pulse in Willy's neck. "Nothing."

"Clear!" Nick yelled as the machine intoned "Press to shock, press to shock."

As Nick shocked Willy a second time, then a third time, Gerry grabbed Ken's shoulder. "Come on, Ken, let's get some water. If they need more CPR, someone else can begin. You can come back after you've had some rest." Ken, Willy's best friend, ignored Gerry's plea. He was prepared to continue CPR when he was needed.

"We need one minute of CPR before we shock again," I said. Ken tried to move his hands over Willy's chest, but Gerry still held his shoulder. "That's an order," Gerry barked angrily. "You will walk away. *Now.*"

Ken glared at Gerry, muttered something, then moved back sullenly. Andy Johansen, another firefighter, got into position and, after Mike and I used the BVM for a breath, began compressions.

Willy had been shocked five times unsuccessfully by the time the Prescott rig arrived at the foot of the long slope. It was almost hidden by the clouds of smoke and brown dust stirred up by cars with flashing blue lights that were responding to the report of a Fairfax firefighter down. Grit covered everything and filled the mouths of the EMTs still working to restore Willy's stopped heart.

As Hugh Washington, the Prescott paramedic, and Prescott EMT Sally Walsh came up the hill, Nick shocked Willy for the sixth time. I quickly filled Hugh in on what had been done.

"Continue CPR," Hugh ordered.

I watched, fascinated, as Hugh worked calmly, methodically, and quickly. Moving to Willy's head, he asked me to stop ventilations, then used the steel blade of the laryngoscope to insert an endotracheal tube into Willy's throat. He taped it into place, attached the BVM to the tube, and handed it back to me. "Squeeze," he said, listening with his stethoscope to be sure that the tube was in the trachea, not the esophagus. "Again," he said as he moved the bell. Listening once more, he said, "Okay, you can continue bagging now." Mike stood up and took the cup of water someone offered him.

Hugh turned to Sally who was opening the IV bag. "Sally," he said, "purge a line for me."

"Already doing it," she said. Quickly she attached a long IV tube to a 250 cc bag of sterile saline and allowed the solution to flow through the tube.

Hugh took a prefilled syringe from the IV bag and turned to me. "Stop bagging," he ordered. He detached the BVM and injected 1 milligram of epinephrine directly into the endotracheal tube. Then he reattached the BVM and told me to continue ventilating.

While Andy and I continued CPR, Hugh took Willy's left arm and tied a latex glove around it, just above the elbow. He wiped the crook of the elbow with Betadyne, tapped sharply, then inserted a needle into the vein, looking for flashback—return bloodflow that indicates that the needle is properly situated in the vein. He advanced the catheter into the vein, pulled the needle out, and attached the IV tubing.

"Epi's been in about two minutes," Hugh said. "Let's shock again." He pulled the heavy adhesive pads from Willy's chest and used his paddles to deliver another shock.

"Still v-fib," he said. "Resume CPR." While I squeezed the bag in rhythm with Andy's compressions, Sally switched to the three leads of the paramedic's defibrillator and Hugh contacted Dr. Margolis in the ER at Fairfax Hospital.

When Hugh had summed up the situation, Dr. Margolis gave verbal orders and Hugh administered lidocaine through the IV line, waited a few moments, then wiped the dust from the defibrillator, checked the screen, and shocked again. "Flatline," he said, indicating to the listeners that Willy's condition had worsened.

"Let's get ready to transport," Hugh said as he gave Willy more epinephrine and atropine. "I've done all I can do here."

While Hugh had been working on Willy, several firefighters had brought a stretcher and a longboard up the hill.

"Okay," Gerry said to the milling firefighters who had been standing around, helplessly watching the struggle to save Willy's life. "Listen up. I want you to know exactly what each of you is going to do so that we don't have any fuckups." Gerry quickly organized the gritty, sweaty firefighters into teams who lifted, moved, and carried. Within a few minutes Willy was in the ambulance and we were hooking up the oxygen to the onboard tank with Sally bagging and Andy doing compressions.

With Hugh, Sally, and Nick in the back, I climbed into the driver's seat and Ken got into the passenger's side for the short ride to Fairfax General. Before the rig pulled away, I looked out through the side window toward the crowd of dust-covered firefighters staring at the rig. Although they knew we would do all we could, most of them already understood that Willy wasn't going to make it. As the rig pulled away, I watched firefighters amble down the hill, milling around, unwilling to leave the scene, as if leaving would be admitting that Willy was gone.

"All for a stinking brushfire," Ken muttered, tears rolling down his cheeks. "All for a stinking brushfire."

A few weeks later, there was a memorial service for Willy. I was a bit reluctant to attend, although I knew I wanted to be there. As I entered the meeting hall at the fire house, Gerry and Ken saw me. "Hey, Ed, thanks for coming." Ken walked up, his eyes red and swollen, and hugged me, pounding my back with his large palms. "Thanks, man. Thanks."

I sighed. Thanks for what? I wondered. We couldn't save him.

As if reading my mind, Gerry said, "It's good to know he had every chance. It's good to know that."

He did, I knew. He had every chance.

In order to become an emergency medical technician, we have to take a course consisting of between 100 and 150 hours of instruction and practice, and then spend time in the emergency room of a local hospital. The amount of time spent in both the classroom and the hospital depends on the state.

In the classroom, we learn how emergency medical situations are supposed to be handled under ideal conditions, which, of course, we never see. The ER time is used to practice taking vitals, to hone our psychological first aid skills, and to learn how the hospital handles patients after we deliver them.

Before he moved to Fairfax, Steve Nesbitt lived in a small town in the Midwest. Although he had the following experience when he was doing his emergency room time at a hospital, unfortunately things like this occur everywhere. Steve tells it like this:

It happened about ten years ago. It had been a quiet evening at a small town suburban hospital ER. The emergency room was empty and the doctor was in the physicians' lounge, watching TV. The ambulance crew that brought in the patient—a black man in his early twenties—told the ER staff that he had been stabbed by his girlfriend and that his vitals at the scene had been within normal range. The crew members transferred the young man to the hospital stretcher, finished their paperwork, and left.

I had almost finished my EMT course and was doing

my ER training, lamenting the fact that I had had almost nothing to do. The man was lying on the hospital gurney in one of the cubicles, surrounded by all the trappings of the ER: oxygen equipment, IV setups, drugs, bandages. He was moaning and crying for his mother. I was anxious to relieve my boredom by at least watching them work up this patient.

As I watched the scene unfold, I wondered why no one came in to examine the youngster. I watched as the nurses hung back, reluctant to approach him. As I listened to bits of their hushed conversation, I gathered that since he was black and had been involved in violence, they assumed that he must be drunk or on drugs or something. They also assumed that he had at least one communicable disease.

They took their time, then one of them pulled on two pair of gloves and cursorily examined his wound, a small laceration in the top of his shoulder, above his collarbone. She checked the young man's pulse and noted the rate and quality on his chart. Despite the fact that he was obviously in a great deal of pain, the nurse decided that the wound was minor—not worth disturbing the doctor's TV program. She quickly moved away from him and returned to the nurses' station.

The young man was in increasing agony, now crying loudly. He was also terrified and complaining that he could not breathe. The nurses stood back and watched him with bored, disapproving expressions. "They always make such a fuss," one nurse said as she sat down in the area behind the desk and picked up her coffee. "The wound is minor and his pulse is okay. He'll wait for a little while." They would let the doctor finish his TV program.

"Please, someone just talk to me," the young man cried. "I'm scared and I can't breathe right."

I was new to hospitals and I had been doing what the others did. But when he asked someone to talk to him,

I went over and, seeing how frightened he was, held his hand.

"My name's Steve, what's yours?"

"B.J.," the youngster said.

"I'll stay with you until the doctor comes in," I said. It didn't even occur to me to question the behavior of the ER staff, to demand that the doctor examine him. I pulled up a stool and asked B.J. about his family, his life, and *Star Trek* in all its forms, a fanaticism we shared. After what seemed like hours, the doctor's TV program ended and he came in to examine his patient.

Then the struggle to try to save the young man's life began.

"We've got a probable hemo-pneumothorax," the doctor yelled as he removed his stethoscope from B.J.'s body. "The thin blade must have entered through his shoulder and penetrated his lung." He turned to me and explained. "His chest cavity is filling with blood and air and one lung has collapsed. He can't breathe." He started to yell for lab technicians, equipment, and drugs. I shook my head. The young man had been dying while the nurses had been drinking coffee and the doctor had been watching his sitcom.

After a couple of hours of frantic activity, B.J. was taken to the intensive care unit. I never learned whether he lived or died, and I never completely forgave myself for my silent complicity in the behavior of the ER staff. I'd like to think that things have changed since then, but I moved away soon after. I never did have to be part of a crew that brought a critically ill patient to that ER.

Pam Kovacs and her crew went on a fire standby late one evening. A few days later she told us about the un-usual situation she got into.

When we arrived at the house on Franklin Street, there were already three engines on location, pouring hundreds of gallons of water on a fully involved, two-story colonial. I went over to the chief who was standing beside a woman in a bathrobe. "Is there anyone hurt?" I asked.

"Everyone's out and uninjured," Chief Bradley said. "This is Mrs. Albert. It was her house."

"Thanks to our smoke detectors, we're all okay," the woman answered.

"But, Momma," a small voice said, "Harry isn't here."

"Harry?" I said, wondering whether I'd have a patient after all. Of all the calls I fear, severe burns is the one I dread most. I have never treated a bad burn, and I hope to keep it that way.

"My cat," the little girl said.

Oh, damn, I muttered silently. I've seen stories on TV where people risk their lives to save all kinds of animals, from dogs to pigs, from kittens to horses. I can understand the strong feelings that some people have toward their animals, but it bothers me when human lives are risked to rescue them.

"Ma'am," Chief Bradley said. "We'll do what we can to save your cat, but I won't put any of my men at risk."

The little girl just stared, tears running down her cheeks. Her mother picked her up and hugged her. "I understand. And you're quite right." She hugged the little girl tighter and said, "Don't cry, Tammy. We'll get another kitten right away."

"But Harry's my baby."

Suddenly a fireman rushed up to me with a tiny shape in his heavy gloves. Reflexively I put out my hands, and the fireman dropped the soot-covered body into them. It was a kitten, but he was so dirty that I couldn't even tell what color he was. His body was limp.

"Harry's dead," Tammy shrieked, looking at the tiny, inert shape. "Harry!"

I touched the tiny chest, immediately covering my

fingers with heavy, black, oily soot. The kitten was breathing but, although I don't know much about the vital signs of kittens, I was sure that the rate was too slow. I could feel the tiny heart, beating so quickly that I couldn't begin to count the beats.

"He's breathing," I said. "And his heart's beating."

The woman just put the little girl down and they both stared at the tiny body lying limply in my hands. "Will he be okay?" the girl cried.

"He's inhaled a lot of smoke," I answered, "but let's see what we can do." I handed the kitten to Mrs. Albert and got an oxygen cylinder and some tubing. I hooked up the tubing and turned the flow up about halfway. Then I took the kitten back and held the tubing so that the oxygen flowed into his face.

"Oh, Harry," the little girl said, shuffling, "please be okay."

For minutes, the limp body failed to react, then, slowly, I felt the kitten's breathing become deeper and more rapid. His heartbeat slowed to what I assumed was a more normal rate. I continued to supply oxygen to the furry body and soon he began to squirm. "I think he's getting better," I said, delighted by the smile that lit the little girl's face.

"Can I hold Harry?" Tammy asked. She reached out and I put the kitten into her hands. I continued to hold the oxygen near his face, and soon the kitten began to lick Tammy's fingers. "He's purring," she said, giggling.

I reached down and touched the sooty body. "He certainly is," I said. I turned the oxygen off. "I think he should go to the vet first thing in the morning, but he sure looks better."

"Thank you so much," Mrs. Albert said. "This was a wonderful thing for you to do." I haven't done much, I thought. But it feels terrific.

"Come on," the woman said to her daughter, "let's find something to wipe Harry off with."

"I've got something right here," I said. I handed the girl a towel and she began to wipe the layers of black soot from Harry's fur.

"What do you say to the nice lady?" Mrs. Albert said to her daughter.

"Thank you so much for saving Harry," Tammy said. She held the kitten in one hand and grabbed the front of my now-sooty shirt with the other. She pulled me down and planted a large, noisy kiss on my cheek. "Thank you."

A man, dressed in a bathrobe and slippers, walked up. "It looks like they can save most of the back of the house. Kitchen's gone, though."

"Daddy," Tammy said, "this lady saved Harry." Quickly Mrs. Albert recapped the situation for her husband.

"Thank you very much," Mr. Albert said.

The Alberts disappeared into the milling crowd of firefighters, bystanders, and gawkers. We stayed for another hour and, thank God, had no other patients.

You know, it's funny. I got as much of a high out of that rescue as I have about any of my others. The look in that little girl's face was fantastic.

Ed and I have been told several CPR stories because both of us are instructors. You've already read about the young man whose life was saved on his porch by the use of the Heimlich maneuver, a skill taught as part of every CPR course. If anyone had known how to perform that simple trick, they wouldn't have needed to depend on the fact that I lived right around the corner.

Time is the critical factor. Let's say that a man has a sudden-death heart attack. Let's also say that the cardiac arrest is witnessed—someone sees or hears his distress and immediately understands what is happening.

With no time lost, someone calls the ambulance and the police immediately dispatch us. The tones go off at headquarters and we drop everything, get into the ambulance, and rush to the scene. We pull up, remove our equipment from the rig, and run into the house.

You can see that so much time has already been lost. Even if the call is right around the corner from headquarters, precious minutes have elapsed since our patient's heart stopped beating. After four to six minutes with no oxygenated blood circulating to the vital organs, brain cells begin to die. Sometimes we can restart a stopped heart, but we can never regenerate dead brain cells. So, unless a trained bystander at the scene has started CPR, the chances of our being able to save our patient approach zero.

Do you remember how, earlier in this book, Tony Piamonte's heart stopped beating in his doctor's office? My crew restarted his heart, but our chance of success was increased tremendously because the doctors had begun CPR immediately.

If you are interested in learning CPR, as those in the following story did, contact your local ambulance corps, the American Red Cross, or the American Heart Association.

Anne Salierno has been a CPR instructor for more than ten years and has taught more than a thousand students. Although her husband rides with a rescue squad in the southern part of the county, she has never been interested in riding an ambulance. When she and I taught a class together about a year ago, she told me the following story.

It was a beautiful spring morning and I was teaching my third class that week. The group consisted of ten men and women who worked for the local highway department, and the class was being given in the meeting room adjacent to the department's main garage. The class was the result of a hard-fought-for, local program to train all town employees in both CPR and basic first aid.

My students had spent the morning learning how to do CPR and the Heimlich maneuver on an adult and had taken a forty-five minute lunch break. The afternoon session had begun with a section on child safety, then we had begun to learn how to do CPR on a child.

"It is important to remember," I was saying, "that a child's airway isn't the same as an adult's." I looked around at my class and noticed that an overweight man in his mid-fifties was looking off to one side, distracted. "Sir," I said, mentally fumbling for the man's name. Oh, yes. "Chip, is anything wrong?" I recalled that the first thing he had done when they broke for lunch was light a cigarette.

"Sorry," he said. "Nothing's wrong. Nothing."

"Okay." I returned to what I had been teaching. "Now, we were talking about a child's airway. You mustn't tip a child's head as far back as you would for an adult." I noticed Chip rub and flex his left arm, and I then looked at him more closely. His face was ashen and he looked sweaty. "Chip, are you all right? You don't look well at all."

"Maybe . . ." With that word, Chip rolled off the chair and landed, facedown, in a heap on the carpeted floor.

"Everyone get back," I said, moving toward the now-unconscious man. I pointed to one of the students. "Patty, call an ambulance and tell them we have an unconscious man. The phone's on the wall in the kitchen. Someone go with her."

"Oh, my God, Chip!" a man in the group yelled. "Chip!"

As the two students left to find the phone, I knelt down beside Chip and slapped his shoulder. "Chip, Chip, can you hear me? Are you okay?" I got no response. "I'll need someone to help me turn him over." I spoke calmly, trying not to panic the other students, many of whom probably had known this man for a long time.

The man who had yelled moved forward. "I'll help."

As we worked to turn Chip on his back, I remembered this man's name. "Are you okay with this, Matt? Is he a good friend?"

"I work with him and I'm okay. I'd like to help. It'll make me feel useful."

"Yeah," another student said. "We all work together. Oh, God, Chip. He's had two heart attacks before, but his doctor said he was fine now. He even asked if it was okay if he took this course."

I put my ear close to Chip's mouth and nose and checked for respiration. "He's not breathing," I said, reaching for the pocket mask I had intended to use to demonstrate breathing devices. I placed the mask over Chip's face, placed my fingers on both the mask and Chip's jaw bone, opened his airway, and gave him two breaths, watching his chest rise with each one.

I then felt for a pulse in Chip's neck and found none. "Matt," I said to the man at my side, "find your spot and do compressions. Just like we did this morning."

Matt slid his hands over Chip's ribs and located the correct compression location. He looked at me for approval. When I nodded, he compressed the chest repeatedly, counting "One, and two, and three, and four, and five."

I gave a breath."

"One, and two, and three, and four, and five."

I gave another breath.

The pair returned from the phone. "The ambulance is on the way."

"Call back," I said more calmly than I felt, "and tell the police to radio the rig that we have a code 99." Patty ran back to the phone.

After about four minutes of CPR, the ambulance arrived. We watched the crew shock Chip's heart several times with no success. "He's flatline," one of the crew members said finally. "Let's get out of here." Quickly, with the help of several of the students, Chip was loaded into the ambulance and it sped away.

Everyone sat in silence for a few minutes then one woman said, "He isn't going to make it, is he?"

"I don't know," I answered, "but it doesn't look good."

"But we began CPR immediately. Why couldn't we save him?"

I switched into teaching mode. "Many of the victims of sudden-death heart attacks can't be saved despite the best efforts of bystanders and medical personnel. The damage to the heart is just too great. But hundreds of patients *are* successfully resuscitated every year. And if Chip doesn't make it, it will be comforting to his family to know that he had every chance. We all did the best we could, and that's pretty special."

I waited a minute. "What do you want to do now? Continue, or are you too upset about Chip? I'll do whatever you want."

Matt was the first to answer. "I want to learn the rest. It felt good to do *something*, even if it didn't work this time."

I continued the class. Just before we finished the course, one of the class members called the hospital. Chip hadn't been revived.

A bunch of us were sitting around the kitchen table at headquarters recently. As usual, the conversation turned to ambulance calls. "I remember one," Jack McCaffrey said, laughing. "Nick Abrams and I were doing CPR in the back of the rig. Nick was ventilating and I was doing compressions. My back was killing me so I asked Nick to change places with me. As we tried to switch, the rig lurched and my elbow caught Nick right in the nose. As he began compressions he realized that his nose was bleeding all over the patient."

"You're kidding," someone said.

"Nope," Jack continued. "So there I was trying to

bag the patient and get tissues so Nick could blot up the blood between compressions. We switched places again so that, between breaths, Nick could squeeze his nose and stop the bleeding.

"And you should have seen the emergency room staff. Were they confused by all the blood on the stretcher."

"I remember one CPR call," Fred Stevens said. "The patient must have weighed over three hundred pounds. We used four bystanders to lift this immense man into the rig. One of the lifters had a huge cigar dangling from the corner of his mouth, but we paid no attention at the time. So, pumping and blowing, we started toward the hospital. 'Does anyone smell anything?' the guy squeezing the BVM asked."

Fred continued. "Soon I started to smell something too, a smoky smell. I was doing compressions and I started to look around. Needless to say, a corner of the blanket was smoldering, thanks to that man's cigar ash. Without missing a CPR beat, we opened a bottle of sterile water and poured it on the glowing blanket."

"No shit."

"Nope. That really happened."

"If you're still collecting stories, I've got one," Dave Hancock said. "It all started with a cardiac arrest at a huge family party. The poor guy was only forty-five. Keeled over right in the middle of the celebration. When we arrived we had to fight our way through loudly grieving relatives, all waving their arms and crying. When we finally got to the patient we started CPR and did what we could."

"I remember that call," Pam Kovacs said. "You guys took the patient out to the rig and I stayed behind with two older family members who were very upset and short of breath. They were seriously worked up: yelling, wailing, and crying. It got worse when the man's wife called from the hospital and said that he hadn't survived. It took almost an hour until I finally got them calmed down and left."

Dave picked up the story. "We were called back later that evening for another family member who had hyperventilated and was having chest pains. I transported him to the hospital."

Pam continued. "That wasn't the last of our encounters with that family. At the funeral for the original patient a few days later, we were called to transport the wife, who had passed out."

"Fortunately," Dave said, "other than the original patient, no one was in serious shape."

Ed's daughter Davida rode with Fairfax until she went off to college. For the moment her EMS career is on hold, but both Ed and I hope, whatever she does, eventually she will go back to ambulance work. She was capable, well trained, and became an experienced member of her crew. I remember her first call as a senior corps member. She tells it this way.

I joined the youth group of FVAC when I was fifteen, partly because my dad was a longtime member of the corps and partly because of the social life. During those first two years I learned the rudiments of how the rig operates and I took a first-aid course. When I became seventeen, I began to ride with the senior corps as a youth group cadet. I took calls and learned my way around.

On my eighteenth birthday, I graduated from the youth group to the senior corps and began my probationary period. I didn't know whether I'd actually take an EMT course because I was on my way to college and I didn't know whether the area to which I was moving would have EMS volunteers or EMT courses. I really enjoy helping people and being able to "do something."

I had ridden a few call-less shifts on Tuesday afternoons after school with Nick Abrams and Heather and Tom Franks. It was really strange riding with Tom, who was a teacher at my elementary school. He hadn't started to work at John Adams Elementary when I was a student there, but he knew all my old teachers. It's almost embarrassing when he tells stories of the goings-on in the faculty room. It was hard to call him Tom and not Mr. Franks.

The klaxon sounded and the radio blasted, "Fairfax police to the ambulance." A call, finally.

"Ambulance on," Tom Franks said.

"We have a report of a serious PIAA on the parkway, Southbound, just before the Route 42 exit."

"10–4. 45–01 is responding."

Tom and Nick got into the front of the rig and Heather climbed into the back. I waited until the ambulance was clear of the garage doors, pressed the button to close them, then jumped into the back with Heather.

"This is your first call in the senior corps," Heather said to me, yelling over the wail of the siren.

I nodded, just a bit nervous. But I had attended to victims of auto accidents as a cadet and felt pretty confident of my ability to follow orders, which, with four on the crew, is usually all I have to do.

When we arrived, the scene was chaos. Bystanders were screaming and crying and I could see a woman trapped in the driver's seat of a blue station wagon. From the flattened and dented roof it was obvious that the car had rolled at least once. I heard someone yell that there were children hurt. Tom, who was crew chief, immediately called for another rig.

As I stood, wondering where to start, a woman ran up to me, assuming from my sparkling white uniform shirt with the Fairfax patch on the breast that I was part of the crew. She was carrying what looked like a pile of clothing.

"I found him on the ground over there." She motioned with her head to the median strip, about forty feet from the wreckage. "He must have been thrown from the car. He's badly hurt and I don't think he's breathing. Do something." As the bundle of clothing was deposited in my arms, I realized that it was a baby, less than a year old.

I had to do something! But my brain was frozen. I had no idea where to begin.

Nick, who had been getting equipment from the rig, saw what had happened, rushed up, and took the baby's limp body from my arms. He positioned the baby across his arm and assessed his breathing. Calmly, without yelling or sounding upset, he said, "He's barely breathing. Get the pede bag. We'll probably need a small airway and the pediatric bag-mask."

Chaos swirled around me as fire engines, police vehicles, and other Fairfax members arrived. Lights flashed and sirens wailed. My mind was alternately a kaleidoscope of images and blank, just a glare of light.

I couldn't remember where the pede bag was and I couldn't get the words out to ask.

After what felt like an hour but was probably only five or ten seconds, someone else, I don't even remember who, ran up with the short spineboard and the pede bag. Nick put the tiny body on the board and together we climbed into the rig, ready to race, with lights and sirens, to the trauma center.

"Did anyone call for the chopper?" someone just outside the rig asked.

"Chopper's on the way for the driver," another voice answered. "But it's faster to just scoop and run with the children."

Children? Somehow, there was another boy already on the stretcher in the rig. Steve Nesbitt, who had arrived when the call for extra manpower went out, was working on him.

Nick put our patient on the crew bench and strapped him down. As the rig started its race to St. Luke's Trauma Center, he wrapped the baby-size BP cuff around the tiny arm and began to take vitals. "Cut the baby's clothes off," he told me, "and check him over so we know the extent of his injuries. Try to move him as little as possible."

It was easier now. I did as I was told. I gently pulled off the child's sneakers and white socks, struggling to keep my balance despite the lurching of the ambulance.

I found a pair of EMT shears in the pede bag and, as I cut the baby's blue overalls and white T-shirt, I looked over the tiny body. No outward sign of injury. I pulled off his diaper. It was dry. I don't know why that struck me, but it did.

Nick turned on the oxygen and hooked it up to the pediatric bag-mask. I saw him point to the little boy's forehead, where there was a large abrasion and swelling. "He's got a serious head injury and his respirations are depressed, about ten per minute. I'll hold the mask and you squeeze the bag gently when I tell you to. One, two, three, now." I sat on the ambulance floor, took the bag, and squeezed. "One, two, three, again," Nick said, counting. I squeezed the bag again.

Time passed. People moved around and at some point someone else took over bagging the baby. I shifted my attention to the side of the rig and looked at the other little body, a boy of perhaps three. Steve had bandaged a deep laceration on one hip and was now cleaning off some of the accumulated blood, grass, and dirt. "Anything I can do?" I asked.

When Steve shook his head, I took the three-year-old's hand, held it, and talked to him. I didn't know whether he was listening to my words, but I hoped that the sound of my voice might comfort him somehow. I remembered a song that I had sung as a child and whispered it into his ear.

"This old man, he played one, he played knickknack on my drum."

We arrived at the hospital and uniformed staff took the baby and the little boy. I watched in fascination as they worked. They were still working on both patients when we left the hospital.

When we got back to headquarters we were all badly shook.

"Fuckin' bitch," Tom said. "It's bad enough not to buckle yourself, but you've got to take care of your children."

I'd never heard Tom swear like that. I'd never heard a *teacher* swear like that.

"The younger kid was in a safety seat," Nick said, "but I heard one of the cops say that he was not buckled. He went out the side window when the car rolled. The older one was unrestrained."

People handled themselves in different ways. Some, like Tom, cursed, Some sat in silence. Heather and I cried. Maybe it's easier for women, who've been taught that it's all right to cry.

"I froze," Pam Kovacs said at one point. "I saw that three-year-old, so badly hurt, and I had no idea what to do." Pam, a longtime corps member, had arrived soon after the rig.

"You froze?" I said softly. Pam nodded. "Me too," I whispered.

"It happens, and you never know what will set you off. It's the worst with kids." Whether she actually froze or was saying that to help me, I will never know, but somehow I felt better.

Over the next few hours, everyone second-guessed him- or herself, just as I did. I mentioned that I hadn't been able to remember where the pede bag was. I knew that it hadn't mattered. Others talked about the things they had done and what they might have done better; they debated whether they should have waited for the helicopter for the children. They tried to learn for the next time. I hoped there wouldn't be a next time but realized that, despite everything, this was still something I wanted to do.

Later that afternoon, Nick called St. Luke's. "The

three-year-old should make it," he told us as he hung up the phone. "The mother and the baby didn't survive. Never had a chance. She died from massive blood loss and the baby had a traumatic brain injury."

That call occurred several years ago, before crisis counseling was available. Now a crisis debriefing team would help us get past the agony that we all felt. At that time, we each handled it in our own way. Dad, Joan, and I talked about it and cried together.

Middle Village is a very upscale, horsey, rural community about twenty miles north of Fairfax. At all hours of the day and evening the roads are cluttered with horses and their riders. Horse farms, stables, and riding academies are everywhere.

Denise Stafford is an EMT with the Middle Village Rescue Squad. I met her a few years ago in an EMT course and she shared the following story with me.

The pagers sounded. "County control to the Middle Village Rescue Squad. A crew is needed for a woman kicked by a horse. A man will meet you at the intersection of County Route 5 and the old electric company right-of-way and lead you in. Call in please."

I radioed the dispatcher and drove down Route 5. As I approached the right-of-way, I saw several other cars already there. "Denise," Pete Marcus yelled, "over here."

I pulled over and got out. As I walked toward Pete, he was talking to a distraught young man, holding the reins of a spirited chestnut gelding. "Denise. You ride, don't you?"

"A little," I answered.

"Let's go," the young man said to me.

Pete explained. "We can't take the rig along the right-of-way. Too narrow and rocky. Mark, here—" He indicated the now-mounted young man. "—will take you to the patient. We'll find another way to get close. Maybe

County Route 456 to Spring Valley Road." Pete handed me an orange crash kit. "Put your radio inside and go with Mark."

I was dazed. I had been born in Middle Village and, like everyone else, I had learned to ride when I was young. I hadn't even been near a horse, however, in more than fifteen years.

"But—"

"She's bleeding bad," the man named Mark said. "Please hurry."

Few words would have gotten me on a horse at that moment, but those pleading sentiments did. I grabbed the crash kit, dropped my portable radio inside, and, with Mark pulling and Pete pushing, I climbed up behind the saddle. Mark took the crash kit so I could wrap my arms around his waist.

Off we went. As we galloped through the scrub and I hung onto Mark's body, I remembered why I had given up riding. I haven't got the thighs or the behind for it. I only weigh about one hundred pounds and I'm five foot five. Each time the horse's hoof landed, my bones and the horse's bones seemed to be trying to be in the same place at the same time. That two-mile ride seemed like the longest period of time in my life.

When we arrived at the scene of the accident, Mark dismounted and helped me down. Sore and aching, I hobbled over to a woman in her early twenties, lying in the brambles at the side of the path. She had ripped her jeans up to mid-thigh and was holding a red bandanna against the inside of her leg, above her knee. Small injury to be making such a fuss, I thought.

"I can't seem to get this thing to stop bleeding," the woman said.

"What's your name?" I asked, a bit annoyed.

"Hillary," she said. "I'm sorry to be such a bother but I'm really not doing well at all."

I noticed that she was puffing, her skin was pale, and her forehead was covered with sweat. As I pulled on gloves, I admitted to myself that maybe they needed me after all. "Let me have a look at that leg," I said.

As Hillary removed the cloth from her leg, I realized that the red of the bandanna had concealed the seriousness of the bleeding. The cloth was soaked with blood and as soon as she removed the pressure, blood began to spurt out.

There was a two-inch hole in her leg on the inside of her thigh about six inches above the knee. I quickly opened three gauze pads and pressed the wad against the wound. It seemed unlikely, but it appeared that the femoral artery might have been nicked. The femoral artery? I thought. Not possible. It's buried deeply in the flesh, near the bone. But whatever was causing the bleeding, it was severe and the hemorrhage needed to be stopped.

"Mark," I said to the young man, "hold pressure on that wound." I placed his hand so the heel held direct pressure over the injury. "Hillary, take this," I said, pulling off my jacket and handing it to the woman, "and put this around you, then lie down flat. I want to take your vital signs."

I touched her wrist and palpated her radial pulse. It was weak and thready. I used my BP cuff and found that her pressure was quite low. I placed the crash bag under Hillary's injured leg to elevate it, then took out my portable radio. "This is portable 35 to the ambulance."

"Ambulance is on, Denise. What have you got?"

"Female in her early twenties."

"I'm twenty-seven," she said, "and thanks for taking off a few years."

"Right," I said. I returned to my transmission. "Female, twenty-seven years old. Two-inch laceration midthigh with heavy bleeding that we can't seem to stop. BP is 100 over 70, pulse 110, respiration's about 24. What are our chances of getting some transportation?"

"We think we can get to you through an old fire break. We've got a county cop car leading us in. He says we should be able to get within about a thousand yards of you. Sit tight and we'll let you know."

"10–4." I put the radio down and looked at Mark. "Is the bleeding slowing down at all?"

"Not really," he said.

"Okay. Let's see if a pressure point will help." I put the heel of my hand against the crease where her leg met her body, halfway between her hip and groin. Pressure on the femoral artery would slow blood flow to the leg and reduce her bleeding.

As I leaned hard, to make conversation, I asked, "How did this happen?"

"Snapdragon reared." She looked at her horse, quietly munching scrub. "I think she saw a chipmunk or something. Anyway, as I fell, Pistol shied and clipped my leg with his hoof. It was that simple. I didn't even realize I was hurt until Mark saw the bloodstain spread down the leg of my jeans."

"Any injuries from the fall? Are you in much pain?"

"I've fallen hundreds of times and this one was nothing. I'd be fine except for this damn leg. The pain's not too bad. But I feel awful. Shaky and weak. I'm sorry I'm making such a fuss."

"It's all right," I said, uncomfortably aware of the way my position forced my jeans against my sore bottom. "Mark? Is the bleeding any better?"

"Yeah, I think so. Should I look and see?"

"No. Don't remove the gauze. If there's any clotting we don't want to disturb it. Just notice how much blood seems to be seeping around your hand." I continued my pressure.

"It's better," Mark said a minute later.

"Okay. See what happens when I release my hand." I relaxed my arm, now stiff and sore, matching my legs and butt. "How's that?"

"Okay, I think," Mark said.

I shifted around and used a roll of Kling and several more gauze pads to tie a pressure dressing around Hillary's leg, leaving it elevated.

The ambulance called me. "Portable 1 to portable 35."

"Portable 35 on," I said into my radio.

"The closest we can drive is about a quarter of a mile. Can the patient walk or ride out?"

"Negative. You'll have to bring the Reeves and we'll carry her."

"10–4. We'll be there soon. Portable 1 is clear."

"I can try to ride," Hillary said, struggling to a sitting position.

"Not a chance," I said, knowing how difficult carrying her was going to be. She had lost a lot of blood, and her face was getting paler by the moment. "I can't take the chance of that wound opening up again and I want you horizontal."

"But—"

"Down," I said with a smile.

Hillary slumped back. I took another set of vitals and saw that her condition was deteriorating. Her BP was down to 95 over 70 and her pulse and respirations were faster.

We talked quietly until we heard an army of people crashing through the underbrush. While Pete spread the Reeves, I counted four other squad members and three county cops. I thanked whatever gods I could think of that I wouldn't have to use my sore, shaky legs to help carry the stretcher.

We got Hillary settled onto the slatted stretcher and covered her with two blankets. The others grabbed the six handles and efficiently carried her across the rough terrain. I don't know who was happier to see the ambulance, Hillary or me.

We drove to the hospital and left Hillary with the ER staff. A doctor told me that she might need a pint of blood and she would have to stay for a day or two until her body recovered, but she would be just fine.

As I soaked my aching body in a hot tub that evening, I wondered whether I would recover as quickly as Hillary.

A Final Word

The following story is from a letter Ed and I received from an EMT in New York. We felt that it was a fitting way to end this book.

Dear Joan and Ed,

I am a member of my town's rescue squad and I've been riding for a little over two years. At the time of this call I had been a member for about five months.

At 10:55 one evening the tones went off for a motor vehicle versus pedestrian accident on the highway near us. Five of us rolled the ambulance and several others who had been hanging around the station hopped on the fire department's heavy rescue truck.

Upon arrival at the scene I was told to get a BVM and the heart monitor. A fifteen-year-old boy had been crossing the highway on his skateboard to get home for his 11 P.M. curfew. The driver of the car didn't see him. When I approached the victim I had never seen so much blood.

The crew chief checked the boy and found that he was in full cardiac arrest. He told me to start bagging while another EMT did compressions. Every time I depressed the bag, blood started to pour out of the boy's nose and ears. That's when I knew he was dead.

As EMTs we're not allowed to stop CPR so we loaded the boy into the rig and drove code 3 to the hospital. In the emergency room the trauma team examined the back of his head and found a five-inch hole. They pronounced him dead five minutes later. He had died of a skull fracture and blood loss. He never had a chance.

Afterward, we were cleaning up when we saw a couple, who I assumed were his parents, enter the hospital. Dressed in my uniform and turnout coat, I was disposing of a bunch of garbage when they brought the boy's father in to see the body. As I passed the entrance to the emergency room, the man lunged for me. He was screaming and sobbing. "Why couldn't you save my boy? It's your fault." It took a security guard and two doctors to get him away from me.

The rest is blank. They tell me I got back into the ambulance and sat down, not looking at anything, just staring. I'm told that when we got back to the fire house I took off my boots and turnout coat and collapsed in a heap on the apparatus floor. My fiancé, also an EMT, came and took me home.

Despite a stress-therapy session, I couldn't get on the ambulance again for three months. All I could remember was that boy's father lunging for me, blaming me for his son's death. It has taken me a long time to remember about that night, but little by little it's coming back to me. It feels better when I talk to people and the story gets easier to tell every day.

Whenever we respond to a senseless death I remember this call. I urge any EMT or volunteer to talk to people about calls that were hard to deal with. Go to any therapy sessions they can. Take it from someone who's been through it. It helps to talk about it, helps the pain and confusion and especially the guilt.

Thank you for listening.

Jennifer

Thanks for your letter, Jennifer. It sums up what all of us go through when we try to deal with a bad call. We cope, knowing that we've done our best. Then most of us go back and try again. Fortunately usually we are able to help our patients, with our medical skills, a kind word, and a smile. And then there's no high like it.

Ed and I hope you've enjoyed our book. We would love to hear from you, so please write. Tell us your story, as Jennifer did, and it might appear in a future book. Our address is:

Joan E. Lloyd and Edwin B. Herman
PO Box 255
Shrub Oak, NY 10588

The Cast

Fairfax Volunteer Ambulance Corps

Radio Call GKL-642
County prefix 45

Emergency Medical Technicians

Nick Abrams—age thirty-four—works split shifts at the local Mobil station.

Stephanie DiMartino—age twenty-one—works in the local Kmart.

Bob Fiorella—age thirty-five—sells insurance and is able to respond to day calls when he's in the area.

Heather Franks—age twenty-four—works in the lunchroom of George Washington Elementary School and goes to college part time.

Tom Franks—age twenty-five—Heather's husband and a second-grade teacher at John Adams Elementary school in Fairfax.

Dave Hancock—age thirty-one—FVAC's Maintenance officer—auto mechanic at a local auto-body shop.

Ed Herman—age fifty-five—publisher and biotechnology specialist who works from his home. Radio call number 45–22.

Pam Kovacs—first lieutenant—age thirty-eight—works part time for a florist. Radio call number 45–12.

Joan Lloyd—age fifty—writer who works at home and responds to day calls. Radio call number 45–24.

Judy Lloyd—age twenty-four—rode with FVAC for four years before moving to the southwest.

Jack McCaffrey—age forty-five—professor at Fairfax Community College.

Sam Middleton—age twenty-seven—city firefighter—rides various shifts as they fit into his schedule.

Steve Nesbitt—age fifty-one—drives a school bus for the Fairfax school system.

Phil Ortiz—age eighteen—became a first responder in the youth corps then, when he became eighteen, he advanced to the senior squad and became an EMT.

Linda Potemski—age thirty-nine—emergency room nurse at Fairfax Hospital and a longtime member of FVAC.

Fred Stevens—age forty-two—electrician with a local construction firm.

Marge Talbot—age thirty-four—CPA with a large accounting firm. Frequently works via computer modem and thus can occasionally respond to day calls.

Jill Tremonte—age twenty—dental assistant with the Fairfax Dental Group.

Pete Williamson—age twenty-five—professional paramedic with an EMS service in the city.

Probationary Members

Tim Babbett—age twenty-three—works for a local contractor—an EMT but hasn't yet become a full member of the corps.

Davida Herman—age nineteen—member of the youth group who graduated to the senior corps as a probationary member on her eighteenth birthday.

Dispatcher

Greg Horvath—age sixty-eight—retired plumber.

Fairfax Police Department

Radio Call ID GBY-639

Officers
Merve Berkowitz car 317
Eileen Flynn car 318
Chuck Harding car 305
Will McAndrews car 312
Stan Poritsky car 308
Detective Irv Greenberg

Dispatcher
Mark Thomas

Fairfax Fire Department
Radio Call ID GCC-905

Members
Mike DeVito
Andy Johansen
Gerry McCarthy
Willy Monteleone
Ken Stavitsky

Prescott Volunteer Rescue Squad
Radio Call GVK-861
County prefix 21

Members
Paramedic Amy Chen
EMT Brenda Frost
EMT Jack Johnson
Paramedic Hugh Washington
EMT Sally Walsh

Prescott Police Department
Radio Call ID GRQ-325

Officers
  Stan Garth car 715
  Mike Gold car 706
  Roy Zimmerman car 703

At Fairfax General Hospital ER
  Dr. Frank Margolis—emergency medicine specialist.
  Kurt Bankcroft, RN—emergency room nurse.
  Rosemary Harper, RN—emergency room head nurse.

Glossary

ALS (advanced life support)—The crew contains at least one paramedic who can perform the life support functions detailed below. See *paramedic*.

ASAP—as soon as possible.

backboard—A wooden board approximately six feet long and three feet wide. It is used both as a body splint to support the patient's body and as a lifting aid. Backboards are also called longboards or long spineboards.

BLS (basic life support)—Crew members can perform only the skills of an emergency medical technician with training in defibrillation (EMT-D), despite their level of training.

BP (blood pressure)—An indication of how strongly the heart is beating. Two numbers are usually given. (See *palp*.) The greater number, or systolic pressure, is the pressure when the heart muscle is contracting. The smaller number, or diastolic pressure, is the pressure when the heart muscle is relaxing. A typical blood pressure might be stated as 120 over 80, meaning 120 systolic and 80 diastolic.

BVM (bag valve mask)—A device that forces air or pure oxygen into a patient's lungs. It can be used during CPR or to assist inadequate respirations.

cervical collar—A hard-plastic, specially shaped bracing device that surrounds a patient's neck to prevent additional cervical (neck area) spinal damage.

closed fracture—One in which the skin is not broken.

contusion—Bruise.

225

CPR (cardiopulmonary resuscitation)—The process of using external means to circulate the blood, fill the lungs with oxygen, or both.

crash kit—A container, often international orange, that contains emergency supplies for an EMT to use when assisting a patient. The crash kit, often called a crash bag or jump bag, contains such supplies as dressings, bandages, scissors, lights, equipment to take vitals, and gloves. EMTs often carry such a kit in their cars. One crash kit carried in the ambulance is sometimes called a megaduffel; it contains oxygen supplies, such as an oxygen cylinder, bag valve mask, oral and nasal airways, and various types of masks, in addition to first-aid equipment.

defibrillator—A machine that can deliver an electrical shock to try to "jump-start" a heart that is in v-fib. (See below.) The defibrillator used by Fairfax EMTs is semiautomatic. The machine assesses the rhythm and decides whether a shock is indicated. If so, it charges and requests that the EMT-D "press to shock." The manual defibrillator that the paramedics use merely shows rhythms on a screen and on a tape. From that information, the medics decide which combination of shock, medications, and/or CPR is indicated.

diaphoretic—Sweaty.

EDP—Emotionally disturbed person.

EKG (electrocardiogram)—A tracing that indicates the electrical activity within the heart's muscle and nervous system.

EMD (electrical mechanical dissociation)—A condition in which electrical impulses in a heart are unable to stimulate normal contractions.

EMT—Emergency medical technician.

EMT-D—An EMT with added training in defibrillation (See above.) Most of the EMTs in FVAC are EMT-Ds.

ER—Emergency room.

ETA—Estimated time of arrival.

FGH—Fairfax General Hospital, the small community hospital that serves the fictional town of Fairfax. In addition to this hospital, down the parkway there is a county medical facility and trauma center.

flail chest—Two or more ribs broken in two or more places. The flail segment, the one separated from the remainder of the rib cage, moves in the opposite direction from the rest of the chest wall, causing severe respiratory distress.

FVAC—Abbreviation for the fictional Fairfax Volunteer Ambulance Corps. It is pronounced eff vac.

Heimlich maneuver—Choking maneuver popularized by Henry Heimlich and taught by the American Red Cross and the American Heart Association as part of their CPR courses. For a conscious person who can't talk, breathe, or speak, the "Heimlich Hug" can dislodge an object obstructing the airway.

hemothorax—A condition in which blood enters the chest cavity from an internal injury. This prevents a lung from expanding to draw in air.

IV (intravenous line)—A tube inserted into a vein by a paramedic, nurse, or doctor to enable the addition of fluid to the bloodstream or the administration of medication.

jaws of life—A gasoline- or electrically powered, hydraulic tool with several attachments that is used to pry metal from around an entrapped patient. The jaws, also known as the Hurst Tool, are usually used to disentangle a victim from a wrecked automobile.

KED (Kendrick Extrication Device)—A brand-name product. The KED is a plastic-covered, vertically slatted jacket used to immobilize the head, neck, and spine of an accident victim in order to minimize additional trauma while he or she is being moved.

Kling—A brand of roller gauze. Long strips of sterile gauze, prerolled and -packaged, that are used to hold a dressing against a wound. Kling tends to adhere to itself, eliminating the necessity for ties or tape.

KVO—Keep vein open.

logroll—To turn the body as a unit, to minimize the possibility of increasing any spinal injury. In order to transfer a patient lying on the ground to a backboard, we logroll him or her.

MAST (military antishock trousers)—Pants with inflatable bladders in each leg and the abdomen that can be pressurized like a blood pressure cuff. Inflation usually slows the deterioration of a patient in shock. PASG (pneumatic antishock garment) is another acronym for the same apparatus. Currently the efficacy of this device is being debated.

MCI—Multiple casualty incident.

MVA—Motor vehicle accident.

normal sinus rhythm—the familiar lub-dub rhythm of the heart. This is the normal rhythm of a functioning heart. (See *v-fib*.)

open fracture—One in which the skin is broken.

OR—Operating room.

oral airway—Technically called an oropharyngeal airway. This curved breathing tube is inserted into a patient's airway to hold the tongue away from the back of the throat and facilitate ventilations.

palp—Short for palpation. Obtaining a blood pressure by palp means that instead of using a stethoscope to listen to the patient's pulse at the inside of the elbow, the patient's radial pulse (see below) is felt while the BP cuff is deflated.

palpate—Touch a patient's body with light pressure.

PCR (Prehospital Care Report)—The report that our state requires us to fill out for every call.

PDAA—Property damage auto accident.

pediatric- or **pede-bag**—A crash bag containing supplies and equipment in smaller sizes to treat children and infants. In addition, the bag usually contains toys and distractions for younger patients.

PFA—Psychological first aid.

PIAA—Personal injury auto accident.

pneumothorax—A condition in which air enters the chest cavity, preventing a lung from expanding during normal breathing.

point-tenderness—Pain felt when an area of injury is touched or pressed.

prone—Lying facedown.

pronounce—The process of declaring a patient dead. In most states EMTs may not pronounce, whereas paramedics may.

pulses—Places in the body where an artery runs between a bone and the surface. Pulses can be felt with the fingertips. The radial pulse is found in the wrist, the carotid pulse in the neck, the femoral in the groin, and pedal in various locations in the feet.

Reeves—A stretcher consisting of a three-foot-wide assembly of six-foot-long plastic slats covered with plastic. A patient can be placed on the Reeves and the unit wrapped around the body. It keeps the spine supported while allowing the patient to be up-ended or carried at an angle through narrow hallways, over rough terrain, or down stairs. The Reeves has handles at each of the four corners and at the center of each long side, permitting a heavy patient to be lifted more easily.

RMA (refused medical attention)—A patient always has the right to refuse our attention. It is, of course, our job to try to convince an ill or injured person to let us help, but sometimes all our persuasion fails.

stairchair—A narrow chair with small wheels on the two rear legs and handles for easy carrying. A conscious patient can be seated in it, belted in, and carried down a flight of stairs or wheeled across a smooth floor.

stat—Immediately. From the Latin *statim*.

supine—Lying on the back, face up.

thorax—The upper area of the trunk of the body, above the diaphragm and surrounded by the ribs. The thoracic cavity contains the heart and lungs. The thoracic spine connects the ribs in the back.

tib-fib—a short form of tibia-fibula. The two bones of the lower leg. Since these bones are frequently broken at the same time, a break of the lower leg is referred to as a tib-fib fracture.

TLC—Tender loving care.

turnout gear—Coats, pants, hats, and boots made of heavy water- and fireproof material worn by firefighters. We in FVAC wear bright yellow, heavy, lined, weatherproof rain and snow jackets in bad weather.

v-fib—Short for ventricular fibrillation. During ventricular fibrillation, the heart's electrical impulses are disorganized and do not cause the heart to beat well enough to circulate blood throughout the body. Unless v-fib in converted to a normal rhythm, possibly by using a defibrillator, the patient will die.

vitals—Vital signs. Several measurable vitals indicate the stability of a sick or injured person. The vitals we measure are (1) blood pressure; (2) pulse rate and quality; (3) breathing rate and quality; (4) the appearance, temperature, and moistness of the skin; and (5) the response of the pupils of the eyes to light.

Stories of True Medicine

Available in your local bookstore.